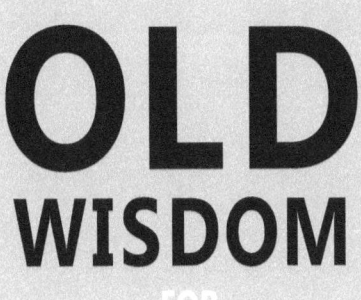

OLD WISDOM
FOR YOUNG DOCTORS

PHILOSOPHY AND FULFILLMENT IN PHYSICIANS' LIVES

GEORGE E. LEWINNEK, M.D.

Old Wisdom For Young Doctors
Philosophy and Fulfillment in Physicians' Lives
Copyright ©2024 George E. Lewinnek, M.D.

ISBN -13: 9798328946421
Imprint: Independently published

Cover artwork copyright ©2024 Jenine Zimmers, (Oakhurst, NJ)

All rights reserved. No part of this book may be reproduced or transmitted in any form or by any means, electronic or mechanical, including photocopying, recording, or by any information storage and retrieval system, without permission in writing from the copyright owner.

This book printed in the United States of America

10 9 8 7 6 5 4 3 2 1

With special thanks to

Susan Tarrant,
without whom this book
might never have been written,
and to

Larry Canale,
without whom it would
never have reached this form.

Table of Contents

Introduction	7
1. Defining Humanism	11
2. Philosophy: Aristotle to John Stuart Mill	17
3. Humanism and Bioethics in the 20th Century	24
4. Challenges to Humanism	37
5. Religions and Humanism	41
6. Hippocrates, Maimonides, and Their Oaths	51
7. Psychiatry and Listening Carefully	59
8. Money Matters	65
9. Cultures and Health Care	74
10. Challenging Clinical Situations	87
11. Five Medical Roles	104
12. Concluding Thoughts	116
Notes About the Bibliography	117
Bibliography	119
Opinions and Acknowledgments	122

Introduction

Values and Medical Practice

I needed to write this book because others in my family did not. My father had studied Latin in school for six years and Greek for three. He read the classics in their original languages, which gave him a better grounding in ancient philosophy than I have. His cousin, Edith Lewinnek Kristeller, M. D., had married Paul Oskar Kristeller. He was a professor of philosophy at Columbia University when I knew him. My father regarded Professor Kristeller's knowledge with awe. English was Professor Kristeller's fifth language. Lecturing in English, he could inspire an amphitheater filled with students, conveying his love and respect for the classic Greek philosophers. I would like to think that he and my father could have written this book, combining their knowledge of philosophy and medicine. Now that task has become mine.

My father had a vision of what it meant to be a good doctor, as did Edith Kristeller, whose thoughtfulness, curiosity, and humility were still evident late in her career when I knew her. For them, medicine was more than a job—it was a calling, to use a term from Dr. Lisa Rosenbaum's article earlier this year. My father's medical calling and his cousin's were expressions of their fundamental values. I learned concepts of being a good doctor from them.

I still had no intention of writing this book until I became involved in a project of other alumni and alumnae of the Harvard Medical School Class of 1967. Before our 55th reunion, the Harvard Medical School Alumni Office had hosted Zoom meetings for us. We enjoyed these social and intellectual events so much that our class leaders arranged to continue them.

One of our speakers was Dr. Arthur Kleinman, author of *The Soul of Care*. A Harvard Medical School faculty member, Dr. Kleinman had done anthropological work with families in China. His scholarly work was poor preparation for the challenges he faced when his wonderful wife developed premature dementia. Her dementia led to her early death. Dr. Arthur Kleinman had a humbling transition from medical caregiver for strangers to medical caretaker for his wife. He described that experience in *The Soul of Care*.

Dr. Budd Shenkin of our class had a similar experience when his wife also developed worsening premature dementia that progressed and caused her death. Our class had trained in the decade after our competitors, the Soviet Union, launched Sputnik, the first man-made earth satellite, in 1957. The national panic at the time was that we were falling behind. Medical schools did their duty and emphasized scientific rigor to us, a rigor often pursued with neglect of humane medical care. Doctors Shenkin and Kleinman learned very little in medical school that prepared them to care humanely for a failing spouse. Budd has organized representatives of our class to correct this deficiency. He started us on a Humanism in Medicine Initiative. Budd's zeal for humanism reflects something in addition to the science focus of our youth: we experienced the idealism of the 1960s.

In the Humanism in Medicine Initiative we learned, to our surprise, that not only have we changed over the years, but that medical schools have also changed. The Harvard Medical School curriculum now includes humanistic material lacking in the 1960s, as does another medical school where I have worked, the UMass Chan School of Medicine. Budd and the rest of us find that we don't need to introduce humanism. It is already offered to you who are students now. Our role is to support efforts already in place.

I joined Budd's initiative but did not understand what humanism is—not in the depth that would have satisfied my father or Professor Kristeller. This book began as my effort to learn more about humanism. The effort grew to include related topics in ethics and other matters that will be important to you who are starting out. I have included examples from my own experiences and the experiences of others that illustrate the applications of theories to medical practice.

In recent years, physician burnout has become a significant problem. Burnout in health care is a large topic. On a major website offering books I found more than 20 books on medical burnout before I stopped counting. Causes of medical burnout include much of what has changed in medical careers, costs, organization, and technology since my generation started our training.

One reason for burnout that this book can address is what the psychiatrist Jonathan Shay called "moral injury." Moral injury is what happens to soldiers who kill in battle, knowing that killing in peacetime is morally wrong. Moral injury also occurs to medical caregivers who are taught in school what is right but then find themselves in the employment of corporations that ask them to do what they were taught is wrong.

My father's values were based on his strong ethical foundation—he always adhered to his values. That was more important to his happiness than greater wealth would have been. He never burned out, although he worked until age 79. You will need your own ethical foundation. You already will have had an ethical foundation by the time that you began medical school. This book will be of use to you if it helps you to review your foundation, perhaps adding to your knowledge, and perhaps helping you to commit or recommit to your ethical values.

Some of you will want to skip directly to the most practical chapters, which are the two chapters late in the book that cover challenging clinical situations and the roles doctors can fill. The basis for these chapters comes early in the book in the three chapters about philosophy, the one about religion, and the one about medical oaths. The book's arc proceeds from these basic values in the early chapters to broadening views in the middle chapters to applications in the later chapters.

I have omitted footnotes in the text, as I discuss in a note at the end of the book just before the bibliography. For those who wish to delve further into any topic, the bibliography will be the place to start.

Chapter One

Defining Humanism

Humanism is a way for people to interact with each other that I observed before I heard its definition. In this chapter we will consider what humanism is and how it can be defined.

Encounters with Humanism

Dr. Francis Weld Peabody gave a lecture to Harvard medical students on Oct. 21, 1925. In it he said, "One of the essential qualities of the clinician is an interest in humanity, for the secret of the care of the patient is in caring about the patient."

Dr. Peabody was the third of four children. His father was a minister in Cambridge, Massachusetts. The fourth of the siblings, Francis' brother John, succumbed to typhoid fever on a family trip to Italy before Francis started college. After Francis completed training that included Harvard College and Harvard Medical School, his travels took him to Germany and China. During World War I he worked for the Red Cross in Romania. Late in the war, Romania allied with the Germans. They expelled all visiting Americans, British, and French. Dr. Peabody fled to Russia, where he witnessed the Bolshevik Revolution.

Dr. Peabody used the word "humanity," not the word "humanism." Humanism is a philosophy. It is a way of living one's life, in or out of medicine, with sensitivity, compassion, and respect for others. Humanistic medicine is but one of its applications. Dr. Peabody had acquired this outlook. His experiences of religion, education, disease, war, death, and civil disorder suggest reasons for his humanism.

I learned of Dr. Peabody's lecture during my second year in medical school. By then, I had already been exposed to humanism. There was an event that occurred in 1946, just before my 5th birthday, at the end of World War II. My father was in Okinawa, serving in the United States Army Air Force as a flight surgeon with a transport squadron. The war was over, but as a medical officer who had never seen combat, my father's priority for transport home was low. My mother's brother, my Uncle Eric, had been in combat. He had served under General MacArthur as we re-took the Philippines. He had been wounded superficially when a bullet grazed the skin over his scapula. He returned to combat and served through the end of the war. Uncle Eric returned home before my father. Home was my grandparents' farm. Uncle Eric arrived with his army buddy Baldy. Baldy had nowhere else to go, I was told. My grandparents took him into their home in an act of humanistic generosity.

The farm was a semi-subsistence farm in northern Wisconsin, where my mother and I had moved to live with her parents when my father went overseas. During the first week that Eric and Baldy were back, Eric had two accidents with Grandpa's car while leaving taverns. My mother expressed to me her disgust with her brother's wildness. Then, my uncle settled down. He and Baldy worked with Grandpa during the daytime. Grandma fed us with food cooked on her wood-burning range. Much of the food came from her garden, her chickens, and the farm's cows and pigs.

I watched one day as Grandpa and Uncle Eric moved the farm bull out of his pen so that they could clean it. Unlike the tame cows and the almost-tame young heifers, the bull was dangerous. He was confused at being asked to leave his pen. It was not clear that he would do it. The two men respected him and even feared him. Grandpa and Eric worked together to herd the bull cautiously out of the barn in a way that suggested their long experience in working together.

The last day that I saw Baldy I heard a commotion behind the machine shed, near the place where Grandpa cut and split wood for the kitchen stove. I went around the other end of the machine shed, near the pig sty, to watch from a perch on the top rail of the fence. Baldy was yelling at Grandpa and Eric. He said that they were taking advantage of him. He worked hard. They never paid him a cent. He had needs. He couldn't even buy cigarettes.

There was rage on his face and in his voice, far beyond what is easy to describe. I thought, "Baldy is having a tantrum. I didn't know that grown-ups could have tantrums."

Near the firewood were an axe, a 10-pound sledgehammer, and a heavy splitting wedge. Grandpa and Uncle Eric had spaced themselves so that Baldy could not reach these weapons. They worked together, herding Baldy as I had seen them herd the bull.

My mother had heard Baldy's rant from the house. Fearing that his red-faced anger might explode into violence, she found me and took me inside to safety.

I never saw Baldy again.

At the time, the name for post-traumatic stress disorder was "shell-shock." My grandparents were not trained in its treatment, but when they recognized the need, they offered a safe, structured, accepting therapeutic environment. I would hope that by the time Baldy left us, he had recovered enough and was strong enough to survive on his own. As I was to learn later, not only caregivers but also patients have responsibilities. There are limits, and Baldy had gone beyond these limits. He had threatened the caregivers' responsibilities to provide safety for everyone else in the household. The message to me was that good grown-ups are generous, but it can get complicated.

Defining Humanism in Medicine

I began my research for this book by looking for a definition of humanism. In Wikipedia, I found definitions, including this: "In the early 21st century, the term generally denotes a focus on human well-being and advocates for freedom, autonomy, and progress. It views humanity as responsible for the promotion and development of individuals, espouses the equal and inherent dignity of all human beings, and emphasizes a concern for humans in relation to the world."

Also, "Humanism is a philosophical stance that emphasized the individual and social potential, and agency of human beings, whom it considers the starting point for serious moral and philosophical inquiry."

The General Assembly of Humanists International in Glasgow, Scotland, 2022, agreed to a declaration describing humanism with four headings:

(1) Humanists strive to be ethical,

(2) Humanists strive to be rational,

(3) Humanists strive for fulfillment in their lives, and

(4) Humanism meets widespread demand for a source of meaning and purpose to stand as an alternative to dogmatic religion, authoritarian nationalism, tribal sectarianism, and selfish nihilism.

The elaborations under these four headings include affirming the worth and dignity of every individual; responsibilities to society; respect for science; enjoyment of literature, music, performative arts, nature, and physical activity; and solving problems collaboratively.

These definitions are not focused on medical applications. Dr. Budd Shenkin, who is leading our class's Humanism in Medicine Initiative, describes humanistic medicine this way:

" 'Humanistic medicine' means many things to many people. It can mean interviewing patients to find out where they're at, how best to reach them, how to be empathetic. It can be befriending patients, even while being a professional. It can refer to adopting the proper stance according to the problem, as indicated by the classic article on the doctor-patient relationship by Szasz and Hollender from (a) active-passivity, to (b) guidance-co-operation, and to (c) mutual participation.

"It can mean becoming wise, as old-time doctors were reputed to be, rabbi-like. It can be becoming attuned to the cycles of life, from birth to death, knowing when and how to intervene and when to let nature take its course. It can be giving advice that is not strictly medical. It can be being able to call upon literature and philosophy as well as science to help patients.

"It can mean being part of a team that works with patients when curing is not an option. It can be helping patients navigate so they can do things they really want to do, when it becomes very hard. It can be caring for the bedridden, turning and cleaning, cheering up, relating, simply being there. It can be tending sensitively to the dying."

Dr. Budd Shenkin wrote this after a life-long career in pediatrics and after his own experiences during his wife's final dementia.

An experience that my son-in-law had suggests that humanistic medical care centered on the patient can turn so strongly to humanism that care is neglected. My son-in-law developed numbness and weakness in one hand because of disc disease in his neck. He sought advice and care from a neurosurgical office. At the conclusion of her examination, the physician's assistant asked, "What would you like us to do?"

My son-in-law was offended. Humanism is fine, but he was in that office seeking advice and care. He wouldn't have been there if he knew what needed to be done. Why was he being asked what to do?

I started my career in medicine when many doctors focused on the technical aspects of medical care first, then on empathetic caring for and about the patient second, and on their own needs last, sacrificing nights, weekends, holidays, sleep, and family life. My son-in-law experienced a relationship with a neurosurgical care provider who may have attempted to provide patient-centered care, placing the patient first, centering on the patient while neglecting care, at least partially. Achieving the appropriate balance between the patient's interests, the doctor's interests, and the caring relationship between the two is one of the challenging subjects of this book.

For the purposes of this book, I will use a definition of humanistic medical care focused on just three words. The definition is this: humanistic medical care includes responsibility, respect, and empathy. Responsibility is what medical care is all about. Respect involves acknowledging patients' inherent dignity and their right, once adequately informed and if they are capable, to make decisions about their care, even if the decisions are not the ones the physician would make. Empathy involves acknowledging patients' emotions as they deal with threatening health problems. These three words—responsibility, respect, and empathy—require the rest of this book to explore and a lifetime to master.

Later in this book, we will consider the work of Tom Beauchamp and James Childress on biomedical ethics. Humanism is ethical; unethical actions are not humanistic. Beauchamp and Childress address four principles of biomedical ethics. The four principles are respecting patients' rights, doing good, avoiding harm, and being just. The technical names that they use are autonomy, beneficence, non-maleficence, and justice. We will consider these principles in more detail later.

· · · · ·

We continue in the next chapter with philosophy, beginning with Aristotle.

Chapter Two

Philosophy: Aristotle to John Stuart Mill

My father grew up in Berlin, where he attended a classical *Gymnasium* for his primary and secondary schooling. When, late in his life, he met another doctor of his generation who had attended Boston Latin School, the two men immediately bonded over their shared experiences. Although they had been educated an ocean apart, their favorite writings had been the same. These two had been taught by a system that regarded Greek and Roman classics as the foundation for modern thinking and the best preparation for leading a good life.

Unfortunately, there is so much to be taught in today's schools that the classics are now relatively neglected. In this chapter, we will help correct this neglect by going back briefly to Aristotle and then advancing quickly to reach John Stuart Mill in the early 19th century. This will establish the foundation for understanding current biomedical ethics, presented in the next chapter.

Aristotle

Aristotle lived in the 4th century BCE. He founded a school in Athens, the Lyceum. He is an ancient authority whose ethics have shaped Western concepts of virtue and heroism ever since. His influence can be seen in old movies featuring John Wayne and Clint Eastwood, and in the lives of Winston Churchill, Eleanor Roosevelt, and Barack Obama, to name just a few examples. These were individuals who each had a personal code. They could resist popular opinion when they regarded it as wrong, while at the same time engaging with the world rather than retreating into a hermit's life of isolation. They led productive and influential lives that Aristotle would regard as blessed.

In Aristotle's *Nichomachean Ethics,* he describes how the concept of "good" is used in so many ways that investigating its exact meaning is not promising. He did investigate its approximate meaning. He wrote that some regard the good life as a life of pleasure, while others turn to public life for a life of honor, and more satisfying still is a life of contemplation. He uses a word that is difficult to translate, *eudaemonia,* for the best sort of life (pronounced "you-DYE-moe-KNEE-ah"). This word combines the Greek root for good, *eu-,* with the word for a guardian spirit, *daimon.* The word *Eudaimonia* suggests the satisfaction of a life blessed by a good guardian spirit. While Aristotle used the ancient word *eudaimonia,* he taught a more modern concept, that it is one's practice of virtues that leads to *eudaemonia,* not the blessings of a spirit.

The virtues that Aristotle taught include courage, temperance, self-control, justice, managing money, honor, and the social skills of friendship, truthfulness, and wittiness. This list suggests the breadth of his thinking about ethics. For most virtues the ideal lies between the extremes of excess and deficiency—the ideal lies at the Golden Mean. For courage, the excess is fool-hardiness, and the deficiency is cowardice. The Golden Mean is not necessarily the mathematical midpoint but may be closer to one extreme or the other. The one virtue to which the concept of a Golden Mean does not apply is justice. There is no such thing as an excess of justice.

In addition to virtue, to achieve *eudaemonia* one needs practical skills and good judgment. The best sort of person does not seek acclaim from everyone but may seek the opinions of other thoughtful people. It is this combination of a personal code, a willingness to ignore popular opinions when they conflict with the code, and, at the same time, engaging in life with skill and judgment that is still admired today.

In *The Art of Rhetoric,* Aristotle wrote that a speaker may sway listeners by appeals to *ethos, logos,* or *pathos*—that is, to ethics, logic, or passions. As doctors, we may wish to sway patients towards a more healthful lifestyle or to sway administrators towards more humanistic programs. Trained in science as we are, we will be most tempted to use *logos,* but our arguments will be more persuasive if we consider adding *ethos* and *pathos.*

Lesley Brown, a Fellow and Tutor at Somerville College, Oxford, notes in her introduction to a translation of the Nichomachean Ethics that in Aristotle, one finds no value in impartiality, no value in relieving suffering and helping fellow man, and no mention of either kindness or cruelty. This suggests that Aristotle's contribution to ethics, as important as it has been, remains incomplete.

Stoicism

The agora was the ancient commercial center of Athens. The Athenians erected a covered walkway with a set of double columns called a "stoa." Here, Zeno of Citium taught a type of philosophy which took the name "stoicism" from the stoa where he taught. Epictetus, who lived later in Italy, taught stoicism. Part of what he taught survives in a handbook, the *Encheiridion,* in which Epictetus teaches, "Distinguish between those things in our power and those things not in our power," and, "That alone is in our power which is our own work, and in this class are our opinions, impulses, desires, and aversions. On the contrary, what is not in our power are our bodies, possessions, glory, and power."

Stoicism can help a patient who has cancer. What is within the patient's power may be to review a will and to plan the best ways to spend what good time remains. These are not the first thing to suggest to a patient who needs consoling, but the time may come when stoicism will be helpful.

James Stockdale was a U. S. Navy Admiral and fighter pilot who was shot down over North Vietnam. He had learned about Epictetus as a student at Stanford University. It helped him survive seven years of captivity, made more brutal by periods of torture and solitary confinement. That was a time for him to focus on what was in his power and what was not. When he was shot down, he said to himself, "I'm leaving the world of technology and entering the world of Epictetus."

Renaissance and Early Modern Developments

The terms "humanities" and "humanism" emerged in the Renaissance. Beginning in the 14th century the European Christian world rediscovered the ancient Greek and Roman manuscripts. Paul Oskar Kristeller, Professor of Philosophy at Columbia University, whom I mentioned earlier, described how first Italians, including Petrarch, and later other great thinkers, including Erasmus in Holland, made these discoveries. Petrarch and others found that Cicero considered the arts pertinent to humanity to be literature, rhetoric, and philosophy. From that time on, these subjects were taught as the humanities.

But then the related term, "humanism," began to be used with a different meaning. During the scientific revolution, beginning with Copernicus, and during the Reformation, beginning with Martin Luther, questions were raised regarding the existence of God. Those whose beliefs did not include God were known as "humanists." The first humanists were atheists, but there have always been and still are religious humanists, so the naming is anything but precise. The religious humanists may be called "theistic humanists." In this book, we are considering humanism rather than the humanities, with no distinction between the atheistic and theistic practices of humanism.

Immanuel Kant was an important 18th century German philosopher. He described and named the categorical imperative. One form of it is, "Act only in accordance with that maxim through which you at the same time can will that it become universal law."

The Golden Rule is similar: Do unto others as you would have them do unto you. This rule is found not only in Christianity, but also in Judaism, Islam, Buddhism, Hinduism, and elsewhere. One difference in Kant's formulation is that Kant derived it by reason. It is not something to follow because it is the will of God. Another difference is that Kant refers to general maxims and to universal law, while the Golden Rule refers to individual actions. In practice, arguments based on maxims and universal law generally parallel arguments based on individual actions.

Later in this chapter, when we get to the four principles of biomedical ethics, each principle can be considered a maxim that could become a universal law. In my training, I heard the question, "How would you treat a member of your own family with this condition?" One's family falls well short of a universal application, but extending a decision from an individual patient to one's family starts one along the way toward Kant's universal laws.

The next philosopher to consider is John Stuart Mill. He was an Englishman of the early 19th century. He became an official in the East India Company and, later in his life, a Member of Parliament, so that in his life he was involved in business, government, and philosophy. His father and friends of his father were utilitarian philosophers. Their basic utilitarian concept was that "actions are right in proportion as they tend to promote happiness, wrong as they tend to produce the reverse of happiness."

The utility of an action lies in promoting happiness. When given the choice between two or more actions, a moral agent ought to choose the action that contributes most to the total happiness in the world. This has come down to us as choosing the greatest good for the greatest number.

Mill also refers to avoiding pain as a measure of utility. His father's friend, John Bentham, included in utility the prevention of mischief, pain, evil, or unhappiness.

In other writings, Mill uses the word "pleasure" as an alternative to "happiness." The greatest good produces the greatest pleasure, but what produces pleasure must be defined, for it differs from one person to the next. Mill gave two definitions. One was to consider that the greater pleasures were intellectual, moral, and aesthetic, and the lesser pleasures were physical. The other definition was that the greater pleasures are those preferred by the majority. Note that these two definitions would clash if a majority preferred physical pleasures and a minority preferred intellectual, moral, and aesthetic pleasures.

In Mill's writing on government, he referred to the tyranny of the majority—individuals, he felt, should be at liberty to do as they wish, so long as they harm no one else. This is a third way to decide what is the greatest good: let the individual decide, so long as they harm no one else.

Mill wrote, "…the only purpose for which power can be rightfully exercised over any member of a civilized community, against his will, is to prevent harm to others. His own good, either physical or moral, is not a sufficient warrant. He cannot rightfully be compelled to do or forbear because it will be better for him to do so, because it will make him happier, because, in the opinions of others, to do so would be wise or even right. These are good reasons for remonstrating with him, or reasoning with him, or persuading him, or entreating him, but not for compelling him, or visiting him with any evil in case he do otherwise."

Mill was liberal, if not libertarian, in this political view.

Current thinking about medical ethics includes balancing benefits and risks, which is similar to Mill's Utilitarianism. It includes respect for a patient's autonomy, similar to Mill's liberal views about an individual's rights. While difficulties occur in defining the greatest pleasures, and this creates difficulties in using individual pleasure as a measure of the good, utilitarianism remains an attractive and useful philosophy.

Mill lived and wrote after the American Revolution. The Declaration of Independence, our Constitution, and Mill's thinking were influenced by earlier liberal philosophers from Continental Europe, England, and Scotland. These philosophers include Jean-Jacques Rousseau, Thomas Hobbes, John Locke, and David Hume. Their thinking is more important today for its effect on our law and government and less important for medical humanism and bio-medical ethics. It would be a distraction for us to consider it in detail, so that it is more appropriate to omit it. For those interested, I would suggest starting with our Declaration of Independence.

• • • • •

In the next chapter, we will turn to developments in the 20th century.

Chapter Three

Humanism and Bioethics in the 20th Century

The 20th century was a time of great excitements and great tragedies, of great deeds and of great villainies. A brief consideration of the century's wars and other events will help us understand a resurgent interest in humanity late in the century and a developing interest in global health.

The Turbulent First Half of the 20th Century

The century began with a proud, aggressive, and short-sighted German nation seeking equal standing with other leading nations. Germany and the rest of Europe entered into a fragile pair of opposing alliances that collapsed into World War I, with hostilities from 1914 to 1918. Germany was the leader of the losers. It was punished by the victors, who demanded reparations. Germany had just begun to recover economically from the reparations when the worldwide economic depression occurred in the 1930s.

At this point, a significant number of Germans listened to Adolph Hitler, who promised them their rightful place in the world as overlords, or *uber Menschen*. This led them first to aggressive diplomacy at the expense of weaker neighbors and then into the full fury of World War II, 1938 to 1944. The United States joined in the response. An alliance of England, Russia, the United States, and others prevented Germany from dominating the rest of the world. Had this alliance failed, all of us might now be an underclass under the rule of German Nazis, for at least some Nazis thought about conquests in North America. Fortunately, the Allies succeeded.

After this war, an increasing number of Americans recognized that our own country was not as classless as the ideals expressed by our founders and that our leaders in the 1940s used as justification for our participation in World War II. That brought the United States into the turbulent decade of the 1960s, resulting in increased human rights, first for Blacks, then for women, and still later for others who had suffered discrimination. The turbulence had political repercussions and a backlash that led to a new division, roughly between the more rural and conservative heartland and the more urban and liberal coasts. This division has been central to our elections in the 21st century.

A slightly more complex summary of the 20th century would add in the rapid advancement of technology. The advances were incredible and of great importance in improving the lives of most people. Unfortunately, progress was uneven. The ethical consequences of advances tended to be neglected, so that the problems with DDT as a pesticide, auto safety, and climate change were addressed only after periods of neglect.

Returning to the turbulent first half of the 20th century, a friend, David Dollenmayer, a retired German professor, introduced me to a line from Bertolt Brecht's *Three Penny Opera* (1928). He wrote within the lyrics of one of the songs, "Erst kommt das fressen, dann kommt die Moral."

This can be translated as, "First comes wolfing down some food, then comes morality."

It suggests that morality is a luxury of privilege. There were well-fed thinkers in the first half of the 20th century, including Bertrand Russell in England and Thomas Mann in Germany, who decried the violence of war and urged a return to ethics, humanism, and the humanities. They were ignored. They were like Don Quixote tilting with windmills. It was not they who were wrong. It was their timing that was wrong. There were too many others who were too passionate about other matters. It was a low point for humanism.

Brecht was right. There is a relationship between having enough to eat and ethics, but it is too simple to say that one is first and the other follows. They can rise or fall together. In the wars of the 20th century, it was ethics that disappeared first and it was hunger and starvation that followed. A farmer needs peace, law, and order to plant in the spring with any hope for a profitable harvest in the fall.

Humanism in the Second Half of the 20th Century

When World War II ended, world leaders committed themselves to avoiding the mistakes made after World War I. They did not demand reparations from Germany. They committed to the United Nations. The United States committed money to the Marshall Plan to rebuild European economies after the war's destruction. A half-century of relative worldwide peace and prosperity followed—not perfect peace and not equitable prosperity for all, but by historical standards it was an exceptional half-century. The United Nations and the Marshall Plan were humanitarian and ethical. This response succeeded, while the more belligerent responses after World War I had failed.

There were 20th-century efforts to promote Humanism—that is, Humanism with a capital H—as an organized movement. At best, these have had modest success. One organization is Humanists International, with representatives from 160 organizations in 80 countries. We in the United States are represented by our American Humanist Association. The American Humanist Association has the slogan, "Good without God." It supports atheistic humanism. It has an estimated membership of 34,000, which amounts to only about 0.01 percent of our population.

Humanism, with a small h, has had more success. Humanism,

along with ethics, is a general concern for today's students in a way that is surprising to those of my generation. In finance, a small number of mutual funds now invest in socially responsible ways. In politics some candidates appeal to voters with humanism and ethics. Some of our recent election results suggest that a majority of our country once again favors humanistic and ethical behavior.

Within medicine, the Gold Humanism Honor Society was formed in 2002. The name reflects support from the Arnold P. Gold Foundation. The Gold Humanism Honor Society has 160 chapters in U. S. medical schools. It gives annual awards to students who are outstanding representatives of humanism in medicine.

Medical humanism in the United States had its own low point. Until some point in the 19th or 20th centuries, science in the United States, including medical science, lagged behind the best in the world. At the beginning of the 20th century, Germany was regarded as the leader in medicine, with France not far behind and the United States lagging. In technology, we had begun to do well with the contributions of Alexander Graham Bell, Thomas Edison, and the Wright brothers. Then, in the late 1950s, Russia was the first to launch a man-made satellite, which they called *Sputnik*. The mood in the United States was that we had fallen behind again. We needed to intensify our efforts in science, including our efforts in medicine. With medical researchers focusing on science, it was ethics and humanism that went out of focus.

In Alabama, the Tuskegee Syphilis Study observed poor Blacks with latent syphilis from 1932 to 1972. The researchers wanted to report on the progress of untreated syphilis. To accomplish this they misled their subjects into thinking they were getting care. It was a terrible failure of medical ethics.

Another incident in science that raised later questions involved Henrietta Lacks, an African-American woman from Baltimore, Maryland. Cells obtained from her cervical cancer in 1951 did unusually well in tissue culture. This line of cells is now known as HeLa cells. She was not informed that her cells would be used this way. She was neither adequately acknowledged nor compensated for this use of a part of her body. In 2023, a lawsuit brought by her heirs resulted in an undisclosed out-of-court settlement.

Unconditional Positive Regard

On the positive side of the humanism ledger, in the mid-20th century a humanistic psychologist, Carl Rogers, developed a person-centered approach to troubled patients. He used the concept of unconditional positive regard. He saw that patients could address their emotional problems best in an environment devoid of threat. This required unconditional positive regard by the therapist for the patient and for the patient's feelings and emotions. Acts are different from feelings and emotions. There were acts that he would not regard positively, but there were no feelings or emotions that he would regard with anything but unconditional positive regard. This person-centered concept has been extended to student-centered learning, and to unconditional positive regard for others in government and diplomatic situations.

The Ethics of Beauchamp and Childress

Also on the positive side of the humanism ledger, Tom Beauchamp and James Childress wrote *Principles of Biomedical Ethics,* publishing the first edition in 1977 and the eighth edition in 2019. They presented four principles: (1) autonomy, (2) non-maleficence, (3) beneficence, and (4) justice.

Autonomy involves respecting the independence of each person. It is a value in both the liberal thoughts of John Stuart Mill and the religious values that we will discuss in chapter five. Beauchamp and Childress point out that for a patient to make an autonomous health decision, the patient must have the capacity to make the decision and be adequately informed. (They use the word "capacity," reserving "competence" for the decision of a court of law.) A child who is 5 years old does not have the capacity, while an adult who is 25 years old has the capacity. Problems arise in drawing a line between the two, between not having and having the capacity to decide. Does a girl who is 16 years old have the capacity when she asks for birth control and does not want her parents to know? In most states, including Massachusetts, she is allowed to give consent to sexual and reproductive health care, but she still requires the consent of her parents for vaccinations. For this girl, the separation between not having and having capacity is not a sharp legal line but a broad zone extending across years.

Note the need for adequate information. Most patients lack the information needed to exercise autonomy when they first visit a physician. Providing information is an important part of humanistic medical practice.

Autonomy can collide with paternalism. Hard paternalism involves the doctor making decisions for the patient because only the doctor has the knowledge, experience, and judgment required. This was more common in my father's day. It is rarer in medical care today but persists in public health. Decisions about safe drinking water, for instance, are imposed by governmental authorities in acts of hard paternalism.

There is also soft paternalism, where the doctor persuades strongly, but the patient still makes the decision. Beauchamp and Childress recognize that patients can benefit from paternalism, especially soft paternalism. Decisions about cancer care can be overwhelming, so a patient may welcome the strong advice of soft paternalism. With overwhelming decisions, patients may want more than soft paternalism and delegate full authority to their doctors. Selecting care after a study of five-year survival rates and complications becomes challenging when it is your survival and your complications that you must consider. When emotions interfere with considering all of the facts, it can be a relief to delegate hard paternalism to one's physician. In such cases of delegated authority, Beauchamp and Childress explain, hard paternalism is ethical.

Non-maleficence is avoiding causing harm to others. Maleficence, which is causing actual harm to others, is distinguished from malevolence, which is the wish to cause harm. (The accent is on the second syllable in both "maleficence" and "malevolence.") Clearly, in most cases, we should avoid causing death, amputation, or permanent damage to any organ, including the kidney, heart, or the ears. There are lesser harms that are temporary, like the pain of injecting a vaccine. Lesser harms can be considered costs. The cost of surgery is not only the money, but the pain and the period of disability during convalescence. The cost of cancer chemotherapy includes periods of inactivity due to nausea, lethargy, and malaise.

Some of the most difficult problems of non-maleficence occur at the end of life. Consider a patient with cancer that has spread to the liver, lungs, brain, and bones. The patient is bedridden, in pain, and scarcely recognizes loved ones. When this patient develops pneumonia, is it maleficent to withhold antibiotics? An argument can be made that a sin of omission is still a sin, so do not omit the course of penicillin. I would prefer the attitude of hospice workers, which is that beneficent management of the process of dying involves primarily measures to lessen pain and increase comfort. Prolonging the dying process by giving penicillin may be the opposite of beneficent. I have reached an age where the way my own death will be managed has become a concern. I would prefer the hospice approach.

Beneficence is doing good to others. The definition of good should be the patient's definition. As an orthopaedic surgeon, I knew that an operation that could restore the ability to do heavy work would mean more to some patients than others—a thoughtful construction worker might want the operation, and an equally thoughtful sedentary worker might decline it. In cancer treatment, the numeric used most commonly when I was in training was five-year survival. Unfortunately, some treatments can make life not worth living. To adjust for this, some now use quality-adjusted life years, known by the acronym QALYs.

When the definition of "good" is the patient's, one assumes that the patient meets the criteria for autonomy—the capability to judge and sufficient information to make the judgment. A question arises with suicide attempts. Has a rational patient decided to end life, or have emotions temporarily clouded judgment, or is this not the decision that it appears to be, but a cry for help? Beneficence is a worthy goal, and so is autonomy, but in suicide attempts, the beneficence of saving a life may conflict with respect for a patient's autonomy.

Justice is the fourth principle. Since there is a limit on the funds available, the question arises of how to spend health care funds. Beauchamp and Childress give the example of a heart transplant, which can save a life. It can cost $1.5 million. Most of those who need a new heart are elderly. Even with a heart transplant, their life expectancy is limited. Is it just to spend so much money on one life when the same amount spent in smaller amounts on many people might do greater good?

Tracy Kidder wrote *Rough Sleepers,* about Dr. Jim O'Connell, who devoted his career to treating the homeless in Boston. This is an area where small investments can make large differences.

Public health is another area where small investments can make large differences. Clean water, sufficient healthy food, and appropriate safety measures have greater effects per dollar spent than the complex medical treatments that many of us spend long years of post-graduate study mastering.

There are small contributions to monetary justice that we can make. Before signing a disability claim, consider whether it is just to the rest of society and ethical for us as respected professionals to sign the claim. It is good to think about the justifications for our fees. Have we accomplished something worthwhile with each visit? Something of value doesn't need to be saving a life. It can be emotional support. It may be a careful follow-up with the goal of quality control. Later, in chapter ten, I will describe a patient who requested surgery about every six months for a condition of his hand. When I recognized the pattern, and at the suggestion of friends who were psychiatrists, I began to see him every three months as an out-patient. With that attention he no longer requested surgery. What support I was providing him was unclear, or whether it was worth our office fees, but what was clear was that those fees were more just than the fees for the earlier surgery had been.

Beauchamp and Childress distinguish between moral obligations and virtues. We are obligated to consider the balance between beneficence and maleficence. We are obligated to respect autonomy and to be just. We are not obligated to be empathetic. Empathy is admirable and praiseworthy but not obligatory. It is a virtue. Morals may also be admirable and praiseworthy, but what distinguishes them from virtues is that morals are obligatory. Virtues, such as empathy, are optional.

No one of the four principles is more important than the others. When a decision involves only a little good and much harm, non-maleficence may be the deciding principle. If the balance is changed to much good and only a little harm, beneficence may be the deciding principle.

There is a relationship between Beauchamp and Childress's four principles and the checklist of three factors for humanistic medicine. Responsibility is the first item on the checklist. Responsible care includes the moral obligations of non-maleficence, beneficence, and justice. Responsible clinicians go beyond these obligatory moral values when they pay virtuous attention to emotional states, but the moral obligations are the minimum required.

Respect is the second item on the checklist. Respect includes the obligation of autonomy, but it may go beyond that obligation to include the virtue of unconditional positive regard.

Empathy is the third item on the checklist. Empathy is not an obligatory moral principle but it is a virtue. Empathy is a reason for relieving pain and offering emotional support for distress. It is only one reason, since relieving pain and distress has beneficial physiological effects, but empathy is a sufficient reason for treating pain.

Global Health

I will conclude this chapter by turning to the United States Peace Corps, founded in 1961, and to global health. During the period between the two world wars, some in the United States reacted to the horrors of World War I by turning to isolationism. During World War II, Americans in uniform went much further than they had in World War I, to remote places like North Africa and the South Pacific. That extended the understanding in this country of how large and varied the rest of the world is. The earlier isolationist sentiments became less common. Young people of my generation were the children of those who had fought World War II. Among us were some who had an eagerness for adventure and an ethical drive to do good; this eagerness and this drive motivated them to volunteer for the Peace Corps. After a brief training, they spent two years abroad in poor communities, helping with development, education, and health.

That same spirit motivated some in medicine to commit their careers to global health. Prominent among them was Dr. Paul Farmer, whose work in Haiti and elsewhere was described by Tracy Kidder in the book *Mountains Beyond Mountains*. That book, in turn, has motivated some of you who are in medical school today to commit to global health.

My experience with global health was limited to three months in 1975, when I served with Project Hope in Jamaica. It was both a wonderful experience and a frustrating one. The project I was to support was to help Professor John Golding at the University of the West Indies establish an orthopaedic residency. That residency would train local orthopaedic surgeons to fill an enormous need on the island. Unfortunately, the ministry in Kingston that had approved the project could not fund it. I found myself not training anyone, but simply working to treat as many patients as possible. With the two of us orthopaedic surgeons from Project Hope, there were then six orthopaedic surgeons on the island to serve 2.5 million people. That meant over 415,000 people for each of us. In the United States at that time, there was one orthopaedic surgeon for every 22,500 people.

My wife and I shopped at a supermarket that always had the same cluster of beggars with limb deformities outside. One of them had had a tibia fracture that had healed with a grotesque 90-degree angulation, so that he could no longer get his foot flat on the ground. Another had had a fracture of both bones of the forearm that had never healed but had gone on to a false joint. If he held his arm horizontally, the forearm folded in the middle with the distal part dangling down vertically. To my eye, the beggars with limb deformities in public places were evidence enough of the need for more care.

One Saturday, I arrived at the University Hospital to find a motorcyclist who had been hit by a car at high speed. He had spent 24 hours in the overwhelmed emergency ward and yet had had no care for a fracture of the pelvis, the left femur, and the left tibia. I was more worried about his head injury. He was only semi-responsive. The chart of his vital signs showed that his diastolic pressure had remained constant while his systolic pressure rose and his pulse fell. That is the pattern seen with rapidly increasing intercranial pressure, in this case, most likely from a torn epidural vessel and an epidural hematoma. The treatment is emergency brain surgery, removing a part of the skull to relieve pressure on the brain and to expose and control the bleeding vessels. I thought that I would need to defer my orthopaedic fracture care until after the neurosurgeons had operated, only to learn that they had already seen him that morning and did not think that they needed to operate. They had left the hospital. All of our attempts to reach them failed in the time that I spent caring for this patient.

While I was arranging the traction for his lower limb fractures, his breathing became intermittent, in the Cheyne-Stokes pattern, and then stopped. I called a code while beginning to breathe for him using a mask and a bag. An anesthesiologist came and inserted an endotracheal tube, with which he could maintain respiration by squeezing the bag. The patient's heart remained strong. In the United States, this patient would go to an Intensive Care Unit, which would be the best place in the hospital for him to be placed on a machine that could breathe for him. In Jamaica, the ICU was overwhelmed. Our patient was less salvageable than the patients who were already there. He had probably already suffered irreversible brain damage. He would not be admitted to the ICU.

I did not want to be there when the anesthesiologist stopped squeezing the bag. Then everyone would wait for the heart to stop beating before sending this young man's broken body to the morgue. It was cowardly of me, but I didn't have the heart for that. I made a lame excuse about no longer being needed, turned away, and left.

I also worked in the Spanish Town Hospital, serving a town just west of Kingston that now has a population of 145,000. Medical students staffed the emergency department over the weekends. They were without X-ray services since the single technician would not return until Monday morning. Without X-rays, they handled about half a dozen fractures every weekend. Using their physical diagnosis skills and their medical knowledge, they were 100 percent accurate. During the three months I worked there, they never said there was a fracture when there was none, and they never said that there was no fracture when there was one. Sometimes, when the lack of funds demands frugal care, skill can replace technology.

Every week we had a meeting of all the volunteers at the Project Hope headquarters. After I had been in Jamaica for a month or so, I had an idea. I discussed it with others at one of these meetings. If Jamaica could not afford orthopaedic surgeons, we could improve care by training bone-setters. It might take a year or two of education, but we could train people to take simple X-rays, to apply casts, and perhaps to inject anesthetic nerve blocks before performing the simpler reductions that would straighten fractures or replace dislocated joints in their original positions. The bone-setters might treat only the fractures and dislocations that were simplest to treat, but that might be half to three-quarters of all injuries. Treating those injuries well would improve orthopaedic health care in Jamaica.

One of the older Project Hope officials patiently explained to me, the most junior person in our Jamaica effort, why my idea wouldn't work. I was proposing something inferior to first-world care. No bureaucrat and no politician in the third world would dare back such a program, for fear of being attacked as a colonialist. I was proposing second-class treatment for Jamaicans, and that would never do.

About 40 years later, at a large, international orthopaedic meeting, I met a much younger man who had begun his practice of orthopaedic surgery in Kingston. He told me that Jamaica now had my bone-setters. They are called, he said, "Physicians' Assistants."

In addition to the needs in the third world, there are the needs of the medically underserved in the United States. You who read this are likely to know already who the underserved are. They are the poor in the inner cities, on Indian reservations, or in rural and small-town America. Their care is limited, and it is getting worse. The town of 9,000 in Wisconsin where I grew up lost its hospital several years ago. A pair of adjoining towns in Massachusetts where I practiced for years, an hour's drive from Boston, and with a combined population of over 80,000, no longer has local obstetrics services. The poor in these communities do not have the transportation to reach good care, for they lack the better cars and money for fuel that they would need to travel to present-day medical centers.

This is not right. These inequities do not meet Beauchamp and Childress's fourth moral obligation of justice. I would implore young doctors who read this to make commitments to help the medically needy in the future. The minimal effort would be financial support of those who directly serve the neediest. The maximal effort is more like Paul Farmer's, serving the neediest oneself. The obstacles to improving global health that I encountered—finding the money and navigating the politics—have persisted and have frustrated many. For those of you with the skills to surmount these obstacles and the commitment to follow in Paul Farmer's footsteps, I commend you and wish you luck and success.

• • • • •

In the next chapter we will consider challenges to humanism.

Chapter Four

Challenges to Humanism

In this chapter we will consider challenges to humanism. These challenges can lead us to a richer understanding of the concept.

• • • • •

One challenge relates to the rejection of God. Not all humanists reject God, but atheistic humanists do, as reflected in the American Humanism Society's slogan, "Good without God." In *The Brothers Karamazov,* Dostoyevsky has one of the characters say, "If God does not exist, then everything is permitted."

The belief, that without God everything is permitted, suggests the view that God and only God forbids and permits. Even the briefest consideration of all the rules that each of us follows suggests the error in this. Families have rules, schools have rules, workplaces have rules, towns have rules, and so forth. Everything is not permitted, even without God. But what about the most important rules, like the rule against killing? A theist can follow that rule because it is God's rule. An atheist can consider the alternatives rationally and conclude that not killing is the maxim that should be universal. For Dostoyevsky's character, God may be the only reason for rules, but for the rest of us that is not true.

A second challenge is that there is nothing in humanism that gives meaning to life. Humanism requires that we treat others with respect, honoring their independence. That is noble, but it is not enough to give meaning to life in the way that striving to serve God gives meaning to life. Christians can strive to serve God and emulate the love and compassion of Jesus. Jews can strive to observe the complexities of the law that God gave in the Torah and that Rabbis elaborated in the Talmud. Muslims can strive to observe the pillars of Islam, including five daily prayers to Allah, alms, fasting during the month of Ramadan, and a pilgrimage to Mecca.

For humanists, consider the philosopher, Corliss Lamont, who was once the president of the American Humanist Association. He included the word "progress" in his definition of humanism. He was concerned with the young and with the future. A humanist can spend a lifetime striving for progress in the present, to educate the young, and to improve prospects for the future. That, I would think, is enough to give meaning to one's life.

A third challenge was offered by Didier Fossin, a French physician, sociologist, and anthropologist. He felt that humanism's focus on empathy and compassion, rather than goodness and justice, is a problem.

In rebuttal, consider the current Senator from Massachusetts, Elizabeth Warren, who started her career with the conservative belief that those who entered bankruptcy proceedings were taking advantage of the system or had been profligate. She believed that they had brought on their own problems. In Fossin's terms, the liberal bankruptcy laws had too much emphasis on empathy and compassion and too little emphasis on goodness and justice.

As a young lawyer Elizabeth Warren studied bankruptcy. She was surprised to find that taking advantage of the system or profligacy were rarely the reason for bankruptcy. It was more often a medical problem or other unforeseeable catastrophe that led to financial desperation. That revelation was the beginning of her conversion to the liberal and humanistic beliefs of her later years.

As a doctor I was never involved in a patient's bankruptcy case.

I was involved in cases of patients' disabilities, where I was asked to document medical disability. There was a spectrum, from claims that were completely fraudulent through exaggerated claims to claims that were completely legitimate. If I placed an overemphasis on conservative justice and rejected all claims because some were fraudulent, I would have been cruel and wrong. If I placed an overemphasis on liberal compassion and supported all claims because some were legitimate, I would have been naïve and wrong. Fossin is at least partly right: ignoring goodness and justice is a problem. But we need to add another part, that ignoring compassion and empathy is also a problem. The Golden Mean lies between these extremes.

A fourth challenge involves other cultures. Professor Talal Assad, of the City University of New York, points out that humanism takes a Christian idea of the essence of humanity and ignores traditions such as those of India and China.

Talal Assad was born in 1932 in Saudi Arabia. He was educated at Edinburgh and Oxford. He was a cultural anthropologist who is now retired as a Distinguished Professor *Emeritus* of Anthropology and Middle Eastern Studies at the Graduate Center of the City University of New York. His work focused mainly on religions, Middle Eastern studies, postcolonialism, and notions of power, law, and discipline.

With this background, Talal Assad would know that humanism is based on Western religions. But that does not mean that the ideals of humanism are wrong or anything less than noble and virtuous.

Asian ideas can be different and fascinating without being improvements on Western ideas. Chinese traditional medicine includes moxibustion or cupping with heated cups to improve blood flow, acupuncture along the meridians of the life force of *chi*, and the idea that medications strong in *yang*, such as alcohol, can be used to restore *yin-yang* balance in a patient with a disease strong in *yin*, such as arthritis. I regard these venerable Eastern traditions with skepticism.

There is also modern medicine in Asia, practiced at levels that have earned international respect. There is a Chinese, Korean, and

Japanese emphasis on being part of the group that contrasts with the Western emphasis on individual achievements. My impression is that this leads to greater humility on the part of Asian doctors, which is admirable, but also less respect for the autonomy of individual patients, which is concerning. Fully exploring this difference would be interesting. As far as I have been able to learn, this difference has not yet been studied, by Assad or by anyone else.

Not all that is familiar is of low value; not all that is different is of high value. I regard humanism as familiar and of high value.

• • • • •

This concludes our three chapters on philosophy and humanism. We have considered Aristotle's *Ethics* and its influence on today's concepts of greatness. We have considered Immanuel Kant's categorical imperative. We have considered John Stuart Mill's concepts of liberty and the utility of the greatest good for the greatest number. With that background, we turned to current concepts of biomedical ethics, with the four principles of autonomy, non-maleficence, beneficence, and justice. We considered global health. We concluded with criticisms of humanism.

The purpose of these chapters has not been to change the values and beliefs that you already have. The hope is that these chapters will lead you to greater knowledge, reflection on what good work is, and greater commitment to your own values.

A sense of doing good work is important. It can be our greatest reward. Consider the stories at the beginning of this book. The two doctors who cared for their wives in their final dementia and my grandparents caring for two young soldiers returning from war with emotional scars all had the rewards of knowing that they had done good work. That reward is not monetary. It is priceless.

In the next chapter we turn to religions, with special attention to humanism within religions.

Chapter Five

Religions and Humanism

In this chapter, we will concentrate on three major religions. These three religions, to list them in historical order, are Judaism, Christianity, and Islam. We will touch on three other religions so that by the end, we will have considered six religions, but even this means omitting other important and interesting religions.

The religions of Judaism, Christianity, and Islam all regard the first five books of the Old Testament as holy scripture. Christians call these five books "the Pentateuch." Jews call these the "Torah." The five books begin with the creation story of Adam and Eve and continue to include the story of Abraham, one of the patriarchs of the nation of Israel. From Abraham these three religions take the name of "Abrahamic."

We will begin with the Old Testament/Pentateuch/Torah because of its common role in these religions.

The Old Testament

I once heard a sermon, I believe by a Methodist minister, which used as its scriptural reference the story of two brothers, Cain and Abel. This story is in the book of Genesis, the first of the five books of the Pentateuch. The story is that these two brothers had a falling out over God's acceptance of their sacrifices. In his anger, Cain slew Abel. When Cain was asked where Abel was, he replied, "Am I my brother's keeper?"

The minister went on to say that we are all the children of God. We are made in God's image, and we are all his children. We must treat each other with awe, respect, love, and care. We are all each other's keepers.

In Exodus, the next of the five books, Moses goes up on the mountain to receive from God the tablets bearing the Ten Commandments. The first five involve man's relationship with God, beginning with the commandment, "I am the Lord thy God." The second five deal with man's relationship with man and are most relevant to humanism. This second group of five commandments are that thou shalt not kill, nor steal, nor commit adultery, nor bear false witness, nor covet thy neighbor's possessions. Whether one is religious or atheist, these are important commandments.

The commandment about coveting is interesting. To covet is to envy, one of the seven deadly sins. Envy may lead the one who envies to unhappiness and the one who is envied to burdensome acts of caution. There is wisdom in avoiding coveting.

In Leviticus, the third book, we find the following:

• 19:14. Thou shalt not curse the deaf nor put a stumbling block before the blind, but shall fear thy God: I am the Lord.

• 19:18. Thou shalt not avenge, nor bear any grudge against the children of thy people, but thou shalt love thy neighbor as thyself: I am the Lord.

• 19:32. Thou shalt rise up before the hoary head, and honor the face of the old man, and fear thy God: I am the Lord.

• 19:33, 34. And if a stranger sojourn with thee in your land ye shall not vex him. But the stranger that dwelleth with you shall be as one born among you and thou shalt love him as thyself, for ye were strangers in the land of Egypt: I am the Lord.

In modern English, these commandments might be as follows:

• 19:14. Do not blame people for their medical afflictions nor laugh at their disabilities.

- 19:18. Be good to your neighbors.
- 19:32. Be good to the aged.
- 19:33, 34. Be good to immigrants who come to live among you, for your families were once immigrants in a foreign land.

A theistic humanist can accept each of these commandments as the word of God. An atheistic humanist can accept them as reasonable and logical.

Judaism

Now, let us turn briefly to each of the three Abrahamic religions, beginning with Judaism. Jewish worship includes family prayers on Friday night, which is the beginning of the Sabbath, and a long service on Saturday morning, including prayers, singing by a cantor, singing by the congregation, reading from the Torah, and a sermon by the Rabbi. The service on Saturday does not need to be in the temple. Most Jews would only require that at least 10 adult members be present, which is called a "*minyan*," although debate remains whether to count among the 10 the women of the faith. The religion has survived persecution and the diaspora that scattered the Jewish people. That the faith endured suggests the robustness of a faith centered on the home and small gatherings.

I once commented to a Rabbi about the feeling of community among Jews. The tradition is that the 12 tribes of Israel represent the 12 children of Abraham's grandson Jacob, his two wives, Leah and Rachel, and his two concubines, Bilhah and Zilpah. I had this sense of that family connection in the weekly Saturday morning services. There was no recitation of the words "I believe," as in the Christian Nicene Creed. There was the attitude, "We are all family. Now, here is the law."

The Rabbi responded, "But before Jacob and Abraham, we were all descended from Adam and Eve."

Later, in a physicians' group on social media, a doctor who was born in the U.S. and was Islamic by birth and choice wrote about a problem. Patients repeatedly asked him, "Where are you from?"

The questioners were never satisfied with his answer, which was a city in the United States.

The questioners pressed him, asking, "No, where are you REALLY from?"

I suggested to this doctor that he answer, "We trace our family back to Adam and Eve. Where are you from?"

This is the family-of-man concept. We are all family, so treat everyone with warmth and respect due to family members. It is humanism, whether theistic or atheistic.

One of the annual Jewish holidays is Yom Kippur, the day of atonement. On this day the faithful confess their sins against God during the previous year. If they confess, repent, and resolve to do better, God will forgive them. The faithful will also confess their sins against another person, confessing these sins to that person. In that case, confession, repentance, and resolving to do better are necessary but not sufficient to gain forgiveness. Forgiveness is granted only if the victim of the sin is willing to forgive.

One of my favorite residency professors, Dr. Henry Mankin, would occasionally advise one of us residents, "Be a Mensch!"

He was using a Yiddish word and a reference to Jewish culture. A Mensch is a person, but more than that, a Mensch has feelings, maturity, and empathy. When one of us in the residency became too scientific and too distant from our patients, he would remind us to be more humanistic. That is when he would tell us, "Be a Mensch!"

Christianity

Next, let us turn to Christianity. Jesus Christ was born in the Jewish world. He built on the teachings of the Old Testament, with a new, or at least renewed, emphasis on humility, charity, mercy, and doing good works. When he was asked by a Pharisee, "Who is my neighbor?" Jesus told the parable of the Good Samaritan.

A traveler who had been set upon by robbers was stripped of his clothes, beaten, and left half dead by the side of the road.

First a priest and then a Levite saw him and passed him by. A Samaritan from a land that opposed Israel saw the man, treated his wounds, and transported him on his animal to an inn where the injured man could recover. The next day, the Samaritan departed, paying for the injured man's stay and promising to pay later for any additional charges.

The Pharisee recognized that the Samaritan was the injured man's neighbor. He was the one who showed mercy on him. Jesus said to the Pharisee, "Go ye and do likewise."

This is humanism, and it is the teaching of Jesus Christ.

St. Paul wrote (1 Corinthians 13:13), "And now abideth faith, hope, and charity, these three; but the greatest of these is charity."

In the Catholic church, there is Confession by a parishioner to a priest. Contrition and penance by the parishioner lead to forgiveness by the priest. Confession, contrition, and penance can be compared to confession, repentance, and resolve to do better on the Jewish holiday of Yom Kippur.

In medicine, we have our ceremonies of confession, which can have several names, one of which is "Morbidity and Mortality Conferences." These conferences may involve a public acknowledgment of a failure to do all that we might wish to do. They play an important role in maintaining the quality of medical care, but as experiences for the doctors, they fall short of the Yom Kippur sequence of confessing, repenting, resolving to do better, and forgiveness. They fall short of the Catholic sequence of confessing, contrition, penance, and forgiveness. There is a greater emotional power in the religious rites then in our medical conferences.

In the 20th century, Liberation Theology appeared in Latin America. Catholic priests in South and Central America emphasized a Christian commitment to concern for the poor, liberation of the oppressed, and equality of all races and creeds. This is humanism within the Catholic faith.

Islam

Next, we turn to Islam, the third of the Abrahamic religions. Despite its size, I know less about it than the other two Abrahamic religions. Worldwide, 24 percent of all people are Muslims. Their great prophet, Muhammad, was born about 570 CE and died in 632. The Sunni branch of the faith has five pillars. The one that relates to humanism involves alms. The other four pillars are the declaration of their Muslim faith, five daily prayers, fasting during daytime during the month of Ramadan, and a Hajj or pilgrimage to Mecca once in a lifetime for those who are able. The Shia branch has seven pillars, adding purity and struggle, and with a different declaration of the faith.

A Muslim woman who worked in our hospital as an Arabic translator told us about her Hajj. She described the experience of kneeling in Mecca, surrounded by thousands of others, each absorbed in the familiar ritual of kneeling, prostrating, and reciting prayers. She said that she could not describe the feelings that she experienced. She fumbled for words to describe these feelings, while the glow in her expression and the warmth of her energy were very descriptive.

Alms should be 2.5 percent of the income of those who can afford it. Muslims hold their wealth as a trust . It is a part of God's bounty. They are obligated to share it.

The holy scripture of Islam is the Quran. The Old and New Testaments are also holy within Islam but are regarded as less reliable and less important. The Quran is an assembly of Muhammed's teachings, with a loose organization described as a web. It is a mixture of rhyming and non-rhyming, of poetry and prose. Recitations from the Quran are part of worship. The combination of poetry and prose aids memorization. Some have memorized the entire Quran and are honored for their accomplishment.

Muhammad and later Muslims, down to today, merged government and religion. Both the Muslim governments and the religion emphasize the authority of the community and of hierarchy.

Under Muhammad, the Muslim world extended throughout the Arabian Peninsula. During the Umayyad Caliphate (661-750 CE), the Muslim world extended west from Egypt across North Africa, across the Strait of Gibraltar to include present day Portugal and almost all of Spain, north through the Middle East to the Caspian Sea, and east across present-day Iran and Afghanistan to present-day Pakistan.

Muslims could be fierce in conquest, and then they could be benign in ruling. They preserved the ancient Greek and Roman manuscripts during the Dark Ages in Europe. They tolerated Jews and Christians within their Islamic towns and cities, at least in most places and at most times. When Muslims welcome guests into their homes, they are gracious hosts who serve selected dates, meat dishes spiced with cinnamon, cumin, and other non-European flavors, and pastries enriched with nuts and sweetened with honey.

Scholarship, science, art, and architecture flourished under the Caliphates. I have an interest in architecture. When I saw the Moorish splendors of a palace in Seville, Spain, and the Great Mosque in Cordoba, I recognized a detail used in the 20th century Salk Institute in San Diego, California. In this masterwork, Louis Kahn collaborated with the Mexican architect Luis Barragan, who had travelled through Spain and France. Barragan specified the wide, shallow water channel in the central courtyard of the Salk Institute that copies Moorish designs.

In medicine, our words "borborygmi," for rumblings of the intestines, and "sesamoid bones," for the small bones in the hands and feet that are shaped like sesame seeds, come from Islamic medicine. Doctors in the Middle East today see an increased incidence of kidney stones among the Bedouin, those nomadic pastoralists who routinely tolerate dehydration in their outdoor life under the desert sun. Orthopaedic surgeons in the Middle East can see an unusual fracture of both bones of the forearm, crushed together by the force of a camel bite.

I dwell on these human details because there are those in the United States who demonize Muslims. These Americans focus on the terrorists from the Islamic world. To judge Islam by the terrorists is like judging Christianity by the Inquisition in Spain. It is not just.

· · · · ·

I will now turn to three stories involving non-Western religions. These experiences helped me understand, respect, and empathize with three cultures very different from my own.

An Oglala Sioux Sweat Lodge

The first story occurred in about 1971. During the Vietnam War I spent two years in the United States Air Force, assigned to Ellsworth Air Force Base in western South Dakota. The base hospital served the U.S. Public Health Service Hospital in Pine Ridge, on the reservation that includes Wounded Knee. I ran monthly surgical clinics in the Pine Ridge Hospital.

A Public Health Service internist my age told me that he had taken part in a sweat lodge ceremony conducted by a Sioux medicine man. The patient was an adolescent asthmatic boy whom my friend had been treating. The sweat lodge was a hut with a fire to boil water and create steam. The boy and the medicine man spent three days in the heat and the humidity.

I had an immediate, dismissive, and thoughtless response: "What that boy needs is your treatment with medications and inhalers, not some old Indian hocus pocus."

"Don't be so sure," he replied. "There is an emotional component to asthma. The boy's family has to be present for part of the ceremony. Important family things were happening in that lodge while I was there."

I was humbled by this insight.

Transcendental Meditation

The second story is that of Herbert Benson, a cardiologist six years older than I am and, for a brief period in my life, a colleague and friend. I heard the story from him around 1978. In 1968, Maharishi Mahesh Yogi approached Harvard Medical School, asking someone to study Transcendental Meditation, a technique that he and his followers were teaching. Benson first said, "No," but the Maharishi persisted until Dr. Benson agreed. He found that within minutes of meditation, the metabolic rate of the one meditating diminished. Hypertensive patients who meditated had a drop in their blood pressure after several weeks. This happened despite the absence of the standard medications for hypertension.

Meditation is practiced by followers of Hinduism and Buddhism. Transcendental Meditation had its roots in the Hindu practice. As Dr. Benson described it, there were four essential elements: first, the repetition of a mental device—a word or phrase, like "Om"—to aid concentration; second, a passive attitude; third, a quiet environment; and fourth, a comfortable position.

Dr. Benson wrote a book about this, *The Relaxation Response*, published in 1975.

A Buddhist Cleansing Ceremony

The third story occurred in 2010. My friend Phillip (not his real name) had a fight with his wife that ended a troubled marriage. I offered to let him stay with me for a month or two while he made plans for his future. I was living alone then and had plenty of room. The month or two that I offered stretched to four months and then six months. It was early in the seventh month when I came home one evening after dark to find that he had committed suicide in my dining room. His lifeless body was suspended by the neck with one of my dog's sturdy nylon leashes. Nearby lay the step stool he had stood on before kicking it away. As he fell, the noose that he had fashioned from the leash had broken his neck fatally.

For the first time in my life, I dialed 911. The police came and then others came to take away his body. For three days I could not live in my house. Even after I returned I found that the house was haunted by my memories. In the middle of the night I had to detour on my way to the bathroom to turn on lights. I needed to see again that the corpse was no longer hanging in the dining room.

The woman who is now my significant other arranged to have a Buddhist priest come to the house. The priest led Susan and me on a cleansing ceremony. We went first to the dining room. The priest lit an incense stick. With it I went around the room, using the rising smoke to remove memories. The priest sprinkled cleansing water. She used a gong and a drum to bring back the noise of joy into the house. At one point, I had to turn and face each of the four cardinal points of the compass in sequence, for each direction has significance. We then cleansed other rooms, paying extra attention to the bedroom that Phillip had used.

The priest hung a prayer flag on a tree in front of the house. It fluttered there for 30 days before the priest instructed me to remove it.

Even though I am not a Buddhist, the ceremony helped me. The house was less haunted afterward. Skeptical though I was, non-believer though I was, there was something in the traditional Buddhist cleansing ceremony that helped me.

I had not become a believer in Buddhism, but it is easier now for me to empathize with those who are.

• • • • •

In the next chapter we turn to the traditional oaths of Hippocrates and Maimonides.

Chapter Six

Hippocrates, Maimonides, and Their Oaths

There are two medical oaths that have been passed down from two exceptional medical doctors. In this chapter, we will consider the oaths of Hippocrates and Maimonides.

Hippocrates and His Oath

Hippocrates lived from about 460 to 370 BCE, about the same time as Aristotle's predecessor Plato. We know Hippocrates from brief mentions in Plato's Dialogues, from a biography written about him two centuries later, and from the Hippocratic Corpus, a collection of 70 medical works bearing his name but almost certainly containing the writings of several other authors in addition to Hippocrates.

We accept that Hippocrates was born on the island of Kos and was the son of a physician. Some of what Hippocrates practiced we still practice today. He believed in the importance of examination, of recording observations, of offering a prognosis, and of being cautious in treatment. He held that diseases had natural causes, dismissing superstitions and the decisions of the gods. He described clubbing of the fingers, a sign of any chronic condition causing cyanosis from a lack of oxygen. He described the physical signs of purpura. He understood that a disease could have a crisis and that improvement after the crisis was an encouraging sign. He distinguished between acute and chronic diseases, and between endemic and epidemic diseases.

In other ways, his practice shows its antiquity. He held a humoral view of disease. The four humors were blood, phlegm, yellow bile, and black bile. When the humors were out of balance because one fell or another increased, disease resulted. That is not the modern view, although we remain concerned when anemia results from too little blood, or when phlegm increases, suggesting pneumonia.

For many conditions he could offer only passive treatment, but he intervened when he could. He used a trephine to drain abscesses of the chest wall. He cauterized hemorrhoids. He used traction for treatment of fractures. He was limited by the technology of his day, but within those limits he used effective measures for a wide variety of conditions.

If you are like me, you heard his name first as the author of the Hippocratic Oath. One translation of it is as follows:

> I swear by Apollo, Healer, by Asclepius, by Hygieia, by Panacea, and by all the gods and goddesses, making them my witnesses, that I will carry out, according to my ability and judgment, this oath and this indenture.
>
> To hold my teacher in this art equal to my own parents; to make him partner in my livelihood; when he is in need of money to share mine with him; to consider his family as my own brothers, and to teach them this art, if they want to learn it, without fee or indenture; to impart precept, oral instruction, and all other instruction to my own sons, the sons of my teacher, and to indentured pupils who have taken the Healer's oath, but to nobody else.
>
> I will use those dietary regimens which will ben-

efit my patients according to my greatest ability and judgment, and I will do no harm or injustice to them. Neither will I administer a poison to anybody when asked to do so, nor will I suggest such a course. Similarly I will not give to a woman a pessary to cause abortion. But I will keep pure and holy both my life and my art. I will not use the knife, not even, verily, on sufferers from stone, but I will give place to such as are craftsmen therein.

Into whatsoever houses I enter, I will enter to help the sick, and I will abstain from all intentional wrong-doing and harm, especially from abusing the bodies of man or woman, bond or free. And whatsoever I shall see or hear in the course of my profession, as well as outside my profession in my intercourse with men, if it be what should not be published abroad, I will never divulge, holding such things to be holy secrets.

Now if I carry out this oath, and break it not, may I gain for ever reputation among all men for my life and for my art; but if I break it and forswear myself, may the opposite befall me.

(Translation by W.H.S. Jones.)

Note the responsibility to refer to craftsmen with the knife for patients with stones. Note respect for patients that included not abusing them and maintaining confidentiality. Note the tone of warmth, sympathy, understanding, and respect. There is much to admire in it.

Portions of this oath are outdated. We no longer swear by Apollo and other Greek gods. A modern version was written in 1964 by Louis Lasagna, Academic Dean of the School of Medicine at Tufts University. Lasagna's version is as follows:

> I swear to fulfill, to the best of my ability and judgment, this covenant:

I will respect the hard-won scientific gains of those physicians in whose steps I walk, and gladly share such knowledge as is mine with those who are to follow.

I will apply, for the benefit of the sick, all measures [that] are required, avoiding those twin traps of overtreatment and therapeutic nihilism.

I will remember that there is art to medicine as well as science, and that warmth, sympathy, and understanding may outweigh the surgeon's knife or the chemist's drug.

I will not be ashamed to say "I know not", nor will I fail to call in my colleagues when the skills of another are needed for a patient's recovery.

I will respect the privacy of my patients, for their problems are not disclosed to me that the world may know. Most especially must I tread with care in matters of life and death. If it is given me to save a life, all thanks. But it may also be within my power to take a life; this awesome responsibility must be faced with great humbleness and awareness of my own frailty. Above all, I must not play at God.

I will remember that I do not treat a fever chart, a cancerous growth, but a sick human being, whose illness may affect the person's family and economic stability. My responsibility includes these related problems, if I am to care adequately for the sick.

I will prevent disease whenever I can, for prevention is preferable to cure.

I will remember that I remain a member of society, with special obligations to all my fellow human beings, those sound of mind and body as well as the infirm.

If I do not violate this oath, may I enjoy life and art, respected while I live and remembered with affection thereafter. May I always act so as to preserve the finest traditions of my calling and may I long experience the joy of healing those who seek my help.

Lasagna's version is not as clear about avoiding intentional wrong-doing, harm, and abuse. It omits Hippocrates' controversial opposition to using a pessary to cause an abortion. There have been discussions since antiquity as to whether Hippocrates opposed all abortions or only the attempts to induce an abortion with a pessary. There are reasons to support either side of this argument. We do not need to decide which side is right. We can move on to note that the rest of the Hippocratic oath contains much to study and to follow, or we can accept Lasagna's omission of any reference to abortion.

There is a Latin phrase often repeated today: "Primum non nocere." Translated, it is, "First, do no harm." The origin of the phrase is not clear. Some say that it summarizes important parts of the Hippocratic oath, while others have found later origins. It is a version of non-maleficence.

When I was in college, I overheard a fragment of conversation in a café in an upper Midwest town. A man who may have been a farmer raised his voice to say, "I AM doing something. I am DOCTORING!"

Having grown up in the area, I knew that "I am doctoring" could mean, as it did here, "I am seeing a doctor regularly."

From the fragment that I overheard, I imagined his story. I imagined he had had a problem significant enough to commit time and money to seeing a doctor. It mattered less that he be diagnosed or cured and more that he had acted. He was seeing a doctor. He had transferred responsibility. He had done everything that he could. He was relieved of the burden. When friends said he had to do something, he could say that he already had. He was doctoring.

That transfer of responsibility for disease and injury was important in primitive societies. It is important today. We in the medical profession have the awesome task of assuming these transferred burdens. I sense the solemnity of that transfer in the oath that Hippocrates has passed down to us.

Maimonides and His Oath

Hippocrates gave us his oath in the 4th century BCE. The next oath that we will consider is the oath of Maimonides from the 12th century CE, almost 16 centuries after Hippocrates. It is newer, but it is now already nearly 9 centuries old. Maimonides was a Jew born in Cordoba, Spain, in about 1138 CE during the Muslim Almoravid dynasty. Ten years later, the Berber Almohad dynasty gained dominance. Laws became less favorable to Jews. Maimonides' family went into exile, traveling to several places before settling in Morocco and later in Palestine. Maimonides was a scholar, studying Jewish, Greek, and Arab literature. He wrote a 14-volume work, Mishneh Torah, on Jewish law. Today, many Jews continue to consult it as authoritative scriptural commentary.

While he was in Palestine, a group of Jews were captured by the Crusaders. Maimonides negotiated the ransom that freed this group.

His younger brother went on a trading expedition to Sudan and India. On the voyage, the ship went down, the brother drowned, and the family fortune was lost. After this tragedy, Maimonides now needed to earn a living. He chose to practice medicine. As a physician, he combined his knowledge of Greek and Arabic sources with his own observations. He became an authority in medicine. He wrote about asthma, diabetes, hepatitis, and pneumonia. Although the word "humanist" was not in use then, he had a humanist's broad education, cultural awareness, and respect for patient autonomy.

This is his oath:
> The eternal providence has appointed me to watch over the life and health of Thy creatures. May the love for my art actuate me at all times; may neither avarice nor miserliness, nor thirst for glory or for a great

reputation engage my mind; for the enemies of truth and philanthropy could easily deceive me and make me forgetful of my lofty aim of doing good to Thy children.

May I never see in the patient anthing but a fellow creature in pain.

Grant me the strength, time, and opportunity always to correct what I have acquired, always to extend its domain; for knowledge is immense and the spirit of man can extend indefinitely to enrich itself daily with new requirements. Today he can discover his errors of yesterday and tomorrow he can obtain a new light on what he thinks himself sure of today.

Oh, God, Thou has appointed me to watch over the life and death of Thy creatures; here am I ready for my vocation and now I turn unto my calling.

Questions have been raised as to whether Maimonides himself wrote this oath. We know that it is consistent with the rest of his work and thoughts.

In the oath God has delegated four tasks to the physician: the responsibility to watch over God's creatures, the responsibility to extend his (the physician's) knowledge of life and health, the obligation to respect God's creatures, and the duty to feel empathy for fellow creatures in pain.

Maimonides' oath contains a version of religious stewardship, a responsibility assumed by some Jews, some Christians, and some Muslims. The responsibilities of stewardship include the responsibility for the world, for humanity, and for the gifts and resources entrusted to us as individuals by the Lord God.

Those who are not religious may feel that they have stewardship responsibilities as members of society. We doctors today have benefitted from those who have gone before us. We owe something to those who will come after us. As doctors, we are stewards for a time of a portion of the health care of our communities. It is a humbling honor and a heavy responsibility.

In another work, Maimonides advised that if one's environment makes ethical behavior impossible, one must move to a new location.

For the younger readers of this book, you will have ethical conflicts. Earning a living involves compromises. Some compromises will be trivial and can be ignored. Select your battles.

Retreat when retreat is the best tactic. Sometimes what seems important to you is not, so get advice from those whom you trust. If the issue is important enough, negotiate. Successful negotiators are flexible enough to consider giving up one important asset if they must, in exchange for getting an alternate asset that the other party is more willing to grant. Change will come slowly, and victories will be partial, so be patient. Recognize that if you leave this position, you commit to the disruption of the move and the unknown risks in the new position. The new position may not have the flaws of the old position, but it will have flaws. Moving involves that risk.

If, after you have considered, consulted others, and negotiated, major ethical problems remain, then leave. Make the move. Adhering to personal ethics is that important.

• • • • •

In the next chapter, we will turn to the special skills of psychiatry that every doctor may find helpful.

Chapter Seven

Psychiatry and Listening Carefully

Medical humanism means engaging with a patient. Of all the specialists, the psychiatrists engage most closely with their patients. There are times when they hear what has not been said. Some of their techniques and some of their diagnoses have been useful to me and will be useful to you, whatever specialty you choose.

Interviewing Techniques

I found four simple techniques useful in clinical care. They involve, to give the techniques simple names, thinking (1) about opposites, (2) about scripts for the visit, (3) about me, you, and us, and (4) about one's own feelings. I will illustrate by considering the angry patient who is shouting and using vulgarities in an outburst that is confusing to you, the doctor.

First, opposites: the opposite of anger may be fear. Is the angry patient afraid of something? Cancer, perhaps, or invalidism?

Second, what is the patient's script for the visit? My script is to progress towards a diagnosis and treatment. The patient's script may be to obtain my signature for unwarranted disability or narcotics. The anger may be manipulative or frustration at unanticipated questions by a patient feigning disease. Or, the patient's script may be to gain relief from emotional distress while I am looking for a physical ailment to explain the distress.

The third technique is the list of you, me, and us. Is the angry emotion because of something that you, the patient, brought into the visit, or is it something that I did, or is it us and our doctor-patient relationship? Has the patient displaced anger onto me that belongs to someone at home or at work, or is it something that the patient overheard me say, or have I taken charge when the patient wants to be an equal partner?

Fourth, I, as the doctor, can use my own feelings as a diagnostic tool. There are times when a patient is not using vulgarities and not shouting, but I begin to feel angry. Our own emotions, the psychiatrists teach us, are clues to what our patients are feeling. It is as if we developed this way of sensing the emotions of those near us as we became social creatures. It is not one of the basic five senses, but we all have this sense. If you make the effort to notice it, you too may find it useful.

Psychiatric Diagnoses

Turning to diagnoses, we will start with situational stress. Examples of this that I saw in orthopaedics include the major transitions in life, including graduations, new jobs, marriage, divorce, children leaving home, retirement, and deaths of loved ones. Preoccupied, distracted individuals had more accidents so that my waiting room could fill with those experiencing major life transitions. Internists see high blood pressure and its complications around these times of stress. General surgeons and gastroenterologists see complications of gastric and duodenal ulcers around these times of stress. As doctors, we cannot change these stresses, but we can point out the role that stress plays, urge caution during stress, provide emotional support if needed, and refer when appropriate to those with specific training and resources in managing stress.

The next diagnosis is depression. I would see depressed patients when the orthopaedic problem was the last straw. They might say,

"Doc, just take care of my back pain, and I can deal with everything else."

Friends in psychiatry suggested that I ask about appetite, sleep, and energy. Depressed patients lose their appetite, have insomnia, and lack the energy to do usual tasks. To complicate matters, not all depressed patients lose energy. There are agitated depressions with an apparent excess of energy. The diagnosis and management of depression may require referral to a psychiatrist.

Related to depression is grief. Elisabeth Kuebler Ross wrote about the five stages of grief: denial, anger, bargaining, depression, and acceptance. In denial, the person grieving over a death may say, "I keep thinking that she will walk through the door." In anger, the grieving person may blame an innocent person—such as the doctor—or an innocent organization—such as a hospital—for the problem. In bargaining, a person with cancer may be prepared to spend large amounts of money and travel long distances for a promised cure, however dubious the facts are. In depression, the grieving person is consumed with sadness. In acceptance, the grieving person moves beyond the loss and returns to engagement with the rest of their life.

Dr. Kuebler Ross had long experience with dying patients by the time that she wrote about these five stages of grief. She has been criticized because she wrote from her impressions rather than from formal studies and formal analysis of data. Her study methodology may have been weak, but her conclusions have proven useful in the half-century since she reached them.

I was told once that patients don't necessarily go through the stages of grief in order. Sometimes, someone who seems to have emerged from an earlier stage returns to it. One patient may skip bargaining, another may vacillate between depression and anger repeatedly, and so forth.

Our culture has a tradition that the widow wears black for a year. Severe grief can last that long, and it can extend into a second year or even a third, with periods of descending into an unfocused, black, bleak place. With time, these black episodes should become less frequent. If they don't, or if other problems develop in moving through the stages of grief, psychiatrists may be able to help.

Freud described the grieving process as retrieving memories one-by-one, reacting to them ("hypercathexis"), and then managing them or letting them go. This process may occur in the fourth of Kubler-Ross's stages, that of depression.

The last condition that we will consider is borderline personality disorder, also known as the emotionally unstable personality disorder. A psychiatrist once told me that if he was consulted because of an uproar in which the nurses were certain the doctors were doing something wrong and the doctors were certain the nurses were doing something wrong, he knew that he would find a borderline personality disorder at the center of the uproar.

The name "borderline" comes from the initial description of the condition as being at the borderline between patients with psychoses and patients who are sane. Patients with psychoses need hospitalization or medication because they are not in sufficient touch with reality to function otherwise. Sane people can manage without hospitalization or medicine because they are sufficiently in touch with reality. Borderlines are between the two—they are partially disabled by their condition, they rarely respond to medications, but they are sufficiently in touch with reality to function on their own outside hospitals. They are not completely in touch with reality but they are sufficiently in touch to function.

One description of the borderline's inner demon is that he or she fears engulfment if another person gets too close and abandonment if the other person gets too far away. "Engulfment" means losing one's independent identity and being engulfed in the identity of the other. I have trouble imagining that fear. The word "domination" comes to mind, but domination, which leaves the dominated one's ego intact, may be less threatening than engulfment, where the engulfed one loses the sense of being an individual. "Abandonment" is easier to understand, except for the frequency with which it recurs in the life of a borderline. The borderline person drives others away but can be unaware of their own role in others leaving them. They blame the others for abandonment and never learn to alter their own behavior. A book by Jerold Kreisman that I found helpful has the wonderful title, *I Hate You; Don't Leave Me.*

There is a Diagnostic and Statistical Manual of Mental Disorders. The fifth edition, or DSM5, gives nine criteria for the diagnosis, five of which must be met to establish the diagnosis. The second one is similar to the engulfment-abandonment fears: "Unstable and chaotic interpersonal relationships, often characterized by alternating between extremes of idealization and devaluation, also known as splitting."

Interacting with a borderline personality disorder patient is like walking on eggshells. One moment, you are a hero and the next, a bum, one moment loved, and the next, hated. You are forever asking yourself, "What did I do?"

You may have triggered one of the two fears, engulfment or abandonment, but you did nothing wrong. The trigger that you tripped was a hair trigger belonging to the patient, not you, and set so sensitively that normal interactions would trip it.

At its worst, borderline personality disorder makes it impossible to maintain a marriage or long-term friendships or to hold a job. Milder forms of the disorder exist.

There are other personality disorders that also fall between normal and psychotic. Borderline personality disorders are in Cluster B, the emotional or erratic disorders. The classification is neater than reality, for many patients have characteristics of more than one type of personality disorder. The diagnosis is best made by a psychiatrist, as suggested by the complexity of the criteria in DSM5.

Borderline personality disorder can cause humanism to fail. Humanistic warmth from the physician can set off the panic of engulfment and can lead to an angry outburst. But then, coldness from the physician sets off the panic of abandonment, so that coldness also fails.

Psychiatrists have difficulty treating borderline personality disorders. Neither insight therapy nor medications have much effect.

The technique of behavior modification has had some success. It is a difficult problem for everyone who encounters it.

• • • • •

This concludes our brief introduction to psychiatry and listening carefully. In the next chapter, we will turn to economics. Money matters will have a great influence on your life, whatever you choose to do in medicine.

Chapter Eight

Money Matters

Economists divide their subject into macroeconomics, dealing with national and international markets, and microeconomics, dealing with single entities, such as hospitals and medical practices. The macroeconomics of American medicine are frustratingly complex and understood best through a history of the system. The microeconomics of any institution where you may work depend on basic documents that will be described in the concluding section of this chapter.

Albert Schweitzer

In my youth, Albert Schweitzer (1875-1965) was considered a saint. He was a devout Christian, a philosopher, a humanist, and a physician who spent much of his life serving the neediest in Africa. Trained at Strasbourg University in religion and music, he learned at age 30 that the Society of the Evangelist Missions of Paris was looking for a physician to go to Africa. He enrolled in medical school, and upon completing his training six years later, persuaded the Society to send him to what is now Gabon, but then was French Equatorial Africa, the country just north of what was then the Congo. He used his college training in music for concerts to raise money. He then went 200 miles up the Ogooué River in Gabon to found the hospital to which he devoted the rest of his life.

Since his time Schweitzer has fallen in public esteem. His fall involved money and bias. Visitors to his hospital in the 1950s found squalor, severely inadequate staffing, and meager supplies. These were symptoms of the hospital's severely stressed finances.

The bias problem arose when he wrote that the African was his brother but his junior brother—a statement that he later amended, but the damage to his reputation had already occurred.

Philosophers have trouble defining good. Businesspeople, accountants, and economists do not. To them, if something is good people will pay more for it, so that price correlates with good. To them, humanism is good if it makes a profit. If people aren't willing to pay more for it, how can it be good? They would wonder, what was Albert Schweitzer thinking? Didn't he do a business plan before going to Africa?

Clearly, there is a gap between the world of money and the world of medicine. This chapter will help you to bridge that gap.

Macroeconomics

A classic of macroeconomics is *An Inquiry into the Nature and Causes of the Wealth of Nations*, written by the 18th-century Scotsman, Adam Smith. He wrote that an individual tradesman, working in a free market unrestrained by government limitations, contributes to the wealth of his nation, as if guided by an invisible hand. Smith was concerned that large organizations would influence the government to pass regulations in their favor. Such regulations would interfere with the efficiency of an ideal market of small enterprises and decrease the wealth of the nation. Such regulations would frustrate the beneficial effects of the invisible hand.

Adam Smith was right that an ideal free market rewards productivity in a way that would contribute to overall wealth. The flaw is that ideal markets are rare. One assumption of an ideal market is that both buyer and seller have perfect information. They never do.

Buyers of stocks in the early 20th century made assumptions up to 1929 that were a major cause of the disastrous stock market crash. That crash and the lack of available lending capital that followed led to the great depression and impoverishment of this nation and others. To get us out of the Great Depression, Franklin Delano Roosevelt used the theories of British economist John Maynard Keynes, who understood that deficit government spending would reinvigorate the economy. That is an important story, but it deviates from our interest in medical humanism and ethics.

The Economics of Health Care

What is more relevant is the evolution of medical economics in our country. During World War II, American factories were running overtime shifts to supply war materiel, but with too few workers, since a significant portion of the population was in uniform and unavailable. To avoid a bidding war for labor, the Federal Government placed price controls on salaries. To get around the price controls, employers noted that benefits were outside the controls. They enticed workers with the benefit of health insurance.

During the war, Blue Cross Blue Shield, with origins in Texas, expanded nationally. Blue Cross was the insurance that paid doctors, and Blue Shield was the insurance that paid hospitals. On the West Coast, a system that had begun in the 1930s became Kaiser Permanente in 1945. To explain Kaiser Permanente, I will use the term "first party" to refer to patients and "second party" to refer to providers. Blue Cross Blue Shield was a third party, working with the first party, the patients, to collect premiums and then paying providers, the second party, as health care was needed. Kaiser Permanente was a third party that collected premiums, but it was also the second party, employing salaried doctors and owning and managing the out-patient clinics and the in-patient hospitals that the first party used.

When the Blues and Kaiser Permanente competed in a community, about two thirds of the population chose the Blues for the freedom that they had to choose their doctors and hospitals. About one third chose Kaiser Permanente for its lower premiums.

As different as the Blues and Kaiser Permanente were from each other, together they established the precedent of employment being the basis for health insurance. They left out the young, the unemployed, and the elderly. That was addressed in the 1960s by John F. Kennedy's New Frontier and Lyndon Johnson's Great Society programs. Medicare, to provide health care to the elderly, was passed in 1965 and Medicaid, to provide health care to the indigent, was passed in 1966. I lived through these times, hearing despair from some in medicine over the advent of socialized medicine as these programs were considered. Once they were enacted, the despair over socialized medicine disappeared as entrepreneurial doctors prospered as they never had prospered before.

From a humanitarian point of view, we now had a comprehensive health care system. From an economic view, there were flaws. Little about the system limited costs. Market forces to increase efficiency or encourage cost-effective care were weak or absent. The medical market was not self-correcting, as it would be in Adam Smith's theory of an ideal free market.

Meanwhile, research and development occurred in three types of centers. In the NIH, research concentrated on the basic science of rare diseases. In academia, research concentrated on the demanding procedures that would attract patients to their centers. In industry, research concentrated on the expensive products that create the greatest profits. Medicine changed, decade by decade, but with this type of research and development, and with no effective restraints from the economics of the market, costs grew. Health care consumed larger and larger portions of our gross domestic product.

Theorists reacted. They were impressed with Kaiser Permanente, which was better able to control costs than the Blues. The theorists developed variations on the Kaiser Permanente plan that they predicted would also control costs. They called these "Health Maintenance Organizations" or "HMOs." A variation like Kaiser Permanente that combined third- and second-party functions was called a "closed panel" or a "staff model" HMO. Another variation was an "open panel" HMO. An open panel HMO was a third-party payer that did not provide care but would contract with independent second-party providers. Once under contract, the providers were considered in-network providers. Depending on how the providers were organized, an open panel HMO could be a group model that contracted with individual medical groups of doctors or it could be a network model that contracted with one or more networks of individual groups, such as all of the staff of a single hospital. Under the contracts, the providers would agree to lower fees in return for preserved or increased volumes. The HMO could decide not to cover care that a doctor recommended if they regarded it as questionable. This would help control costs. The first parties, the patients, would be restricted to in-network providers unless they were willing to pay a penalty for an out-of-network provider. The patients were also restricted to approved care unless they were willing to pay out-of-pocket.

The law under which these new HMOs functioned was passed in 1973, during Richard Nixon's presidency. A provision of the law protected HMOs from litigation. To an outsider, the HMOs appeared to be practicing medicine when they decided which care and which procedures were covered. Practicing medicine would have made them responsible for any harm. To the legal community, the HMOs were only deciding which procedures would be paid for, and the doctors who actually practiced medicine were completely free to proceed without being paid. The patients were completely free to pay out-of-pocket. The HMO was, the argument went, not practicing medicine and was not legally responsible for any harms. They could not be sued for malpractice.

Almost as soon as the HMOs were introduced a game began. The game was that providers searched for loopholes in the regulations that would allow them to bill more while the HMOs closed loopholes almost as fast as they were found by imposing more and more regulations. The regulations became a complex labyrinth that could be negotiated only by a growing bureaucracy of expensive medical billing specialists, and even these specialists subspecialized so that orthopaedic billing specialists did not understand the complexities of billing in any other specialty.

The HMO-based market forces that were supposed to control costs did not work, or at least they did not work as well as planned. In my youth, health care was about 5 percent of the U.S. gross domestic product. In 2022 it was 16.6 percent. It is a higher portion of GDP in this country than in any other developed country. Part of the growth in cost paid for expanding and expensive new technology, including imaging and endoscopic surgery. This is not the whole explanation, for these expensive new technologies are used in other countries with less growth in their medical expenses. Defenders of the changes in our system told me that our prices would have grown even faster had the HMOs not been expanded in 1973.

In the 1990s, Hillary Clinton tried to do something to improve our medical system. She convened a National Health Reform task force in Washington in 1993. Its task was to improve the quality of medical care, broaden coverage, and control costs. This is a seemingly impossible task, for costs move in the wrong direction when quality increases or coverage broadens. The task force did come up with a plan, Hillary Care, that did not get support in either the Senate or the House of Representatives. The opposition from organized medicine was too strong.

It was clear to many that something needed to be done, and efforts continued. Almost a generation later and with the backing of then-President Barrack Obama, the Affordable Care Act, known as Obamacare, was passed in 2010. It went into effect in 2014, delayed for political reasons. It broadened coverage. It allowed patients with pre-existing conditions to change insurers. These were significant improvements.

Still, problems remain. In Obama's campaign platform in 2008, one section had supported research and development of cost-effective medical care. This is appealing since increasing efficiency is a way to improve quality and broaden coverage without raising costs. President Obama had enough political difficulty passing the Affordable Care Act. He never got to his platform's proposed measures regarding the research and development of cost-effective medical care. We continue to have the most expensive medical system in the world and yet lag behind other developed countries on measures of quality, such as infant mortality.

Returning to economic theory, those who admire Adam Smith would look to an ideal market to strike the best balance between quality, coverage, and costs. Unfortunately, the ideal market requires perfect knowledge and complete freedom of choice. Both are lacking in our less-than-ideal world. Patients lock into an insurance plan early in their adult life when they start working. Late in life, when they begin to need care, they discover limitations to the low-price plan they had chosen, but now that they have a disease it is difficult or impossible to change plans. (To its credit, the Affordable Care Act addresses this problem.)

On the provider side, Adam Smith would say that workers will move to the best-paying jobs. Doctors who become established in one locality are hesitant to move, even if their income falls. It is only when this underpaid generation retires that the problem is revealed. New doctors decline to move in. Shortages develop. John Maynard Keynes describes this delayed effect as stickiness in the labor market.

Bright, capable, idealistic public health school thinkers have been wrestling with problems of inefficiencies in the health care market system throughout my life. Great problems remain.

I find all of this discouraging. But then, I have lived through many changes, only a few of which have been successful. There has always been a place for doctors who take good care of their patients. I would suggest to young doctors that you focus on that. Taking good care of patients is the honorable thing to do. It can be the most satisfying thing to do. It is the most practical thing to do, for delivering the needed care provides a measure of job security. The changes in health care policy are not under your control. Providing good care to your patients is under your control. Do it if you value job security.

Microeconomics

Let us now turn to microeconomics, the economics of the organizations where you will likely find employment. There are three microeconomic documents to know about: balance sheets, cash-flow statements, and business plans.

A balance sheet uses a basic accounting formula—assets minus liabilities equals net worth. Assets are holdings of value. Those holdings include cash, endowments, buildings, equipment, and accounts receivable for services already delivered but not yet paid for. The accounts receivable may be the largest asset of a group practice. Some assets have fixed dollar values, while others, such as aging equipment and buildings, are estimates that can be fudged in ways that are invisible to most of us.

Liabilities are claims that others have against the organization's assets. These liabilities include hospital bonds, group practice loans, and accounts payable for items that the organization bought but has not yet paid for.

The difference between assets and liabilities is the net worth of the organization. The net worth is the bottom line on the balance sheet. Financial analysts will study changes in balance sheets over five-year spans or longer. They look for stability or growth in net worth. They want an explanation of loan balance increases. Increasing loan balances may mean a struggling organization that cannot live within its means or it may mean a thriving and growing organization making sound business investments. The dry numbers on balance sheets are suggestions to the analyst of interesting stories.

The cash flow statement uses another formula: cash in minus cash out equals the increment in cash on hand. Organizations have entered bankruptcy despite robust balance sheets when cash in was inadequate to fund cash out, the money drawer was empty, and no loans were available to keep the organization in business. Cash flow statements may indicate how partners in a group practice divide profits and whether a senior partner has begun to slow down. Here again, the dry numbers may tell interesting stories.

These first two documents look back. If you propose a new humanistic program, an administrator will look forward by developing a business plan that estimates future cash in, future cash out, and the accumulating deficit or profit, month-by-month, over a period of several years. A careful administrator may do a second and perhaps a third business plan. The first plan will be with the expected growth of the new program. If that shows an eventual profit, care requires a second plan in case the new program does somewhat worse than expected. If the somewhat-worse-than-expected estimates are discouraging, doing a third plan may be worthwhile. The third plan will assume that the new program does somewhat better than expected. If the profits in the best case are exceptional, the administrator may consider taking a chance, known as rolling the dice. Most administrators are cautious and don't like rolling the dice.

If the administrator's business plans for your program are unfavorable, you might suggest that the administrator broaden the focus. A humanistic program can create goodwill. Goodwill is an asset that may appear to have no dollar value now, but it has a value in future earnings. Accountants can put an estimated present value on future earnings. Also, not focusing on humanism leaves a hospital vulnerable to competitors, especially those who compete on the borders of your hospital's service area. There is value in competing effectively. There is risk in not competing effectively.

The administrator with whom you are talking may need to justify your program to a committee. You have now given this administrator the arguments about future value and goodwill that may carry the day. Good luck!

• • • • •

This concludes our introduction to medical economics. In the next chapter, we will consider the variety of national cultures that doctors in the United States may encounter.

Chapter Nine

Cultures and Health Care

Cultural sensitivity is a part of humanism as defined by Corliss Lamont, a past president of the American Humanism Association. While every patient is an individual and a minority of one, they have been influenced by the culture in which they have lived. Understanding a patient's culture will help you engage with them.

I was more than halfway through my career when my hospital held its first mandatory cultural sensitivity training session. Our training session presented lists and definitions. Cultural sensitivity, the presenter told us, was comprised of the following:

(1) a diplomatic stance,
(2) cultural learning,
(3) cultural reasoning, and
(4) intercultural interaction.

I knew that there were doctors on our staff who demeaned our community's immigrants. This training did not change their views.

My hospital's training session on cultural sensitivity used deductive reasoning or reasoning from general principles to specific applications, of the sort that we all used in geometry. I learned about cultures a different way. What follows is a view of cultural sensitivity built up inductively, proceeding from specifics to general principles. We will start with specifics that can be learned from books.

A Few Books on Culture and Medicine

The first book for us to consider is *Childhood and Society* by Erik Erikson. Erikson began psychiatric training under Anna Freud and added his own anthropological view. He studied indigenous American societies in order to trace the emotional development of their children. One society was the Lakota Sioux. This society had adapted to the buffalo hunt. It took tribal cooperation to kill a buffalo, and it took the tribe eating together to consume the huge animal before the meat spoiled. Group cooperation was more important than individual achievement.

From 1970 to 1972, part of my practice was with the Lakota Sioux residents of the Pine Ridge reservation in South Dakota, a reservation that Dr. Erikson had visited. It is the home for the tribe once led by the great chiefs Sitting Bull and Red Cloud. On the reservation the Lakota live in poverty in the comfort of a culture that continues their tribe's earlier pattern, where competition within the group is discouraged, and mutual support is encouraged. Off the reservation they might travel to Minneapolis, St. Paul, or Denver for jobs that paid well, but where the culture was an alien combination of individualism and competition. Many Lakota tried that for a few years and then returned to the reservation, poorer in possessions but richer in cultural comfort.

One of my first Lakota patients was Laurence Little Hawk (I have changed his name). I helped him through an acute attack of pancreatitis. When I drew back the bedclothes to examine him, I found that his swollen scrotum looked like a small, ecchymotic melon. I blurted out, "What's that?"

"A black widow spider bite, Doc. Haven't you ever seen one before?"

I hadn't, so Mr. Little Hawk taught me. The spiders live in the outhouses under the seats. They don't like intrusions hanging down into their space. Mr. Little Hawk predicted correctly that the spider bite would heal with no need for my medical care.

His choice of life on the reservation, including outhouses and black widow spiders, seemed inexplicably impoverished to some of my colleagues. However, it was a choice that deserved honor and respect. It was a part of his culture. The reservation with its poverty was a place of cooperation and mutual support among family, friends, and neighbors. Understanding that was a step toward respect and empathy.

A second book to consider is Anne Fadiman's *The Spirit Catches You and You Fall Down: A Hmong Child, Her American Doctors, and the Collision of Two Cultures*. The Hmong were hills-people who cooperated with our Central Intelligence Agency in the Vietnam War. They fled from the advancing North Vietnamese when the U.S. withdrew from Vietnam, and many emigrated to the United States. The Hmong child at the center of this story was Lia, born in Merced, California. She had a severe form of childhood epilepsy. The Hmong explanation of a seizure is the title of the book: the spirit catches you and you fall down.

The family practice residents who cared for Lia had our medical explanation. There is a focus in the brain that causes the seizure. They treated Lia with anti-seizure medications to quiet the focus, and when the seizures continued, they increased the doses. When that didn't work, they found that the medications had not been given as prescribed. That was child abuse. They had the courts take Lia away from her parents.

The foster mother who received Lia allowed Lia's mother to visit. The interactions the foster mother observed convinced her that no abuse had occurred. Eventually, the miscarriage of justice was reversed, and Lia was returned to her parents, but by that time, the underlying disorder had progressed despite medications. An episode of status epilepticus led to irreversible brain damage.

The treating doctors had given Lia's parents a graduated test tube to measure the liquid medication. Lia's illiterate parents could not read it. That was a failure of cross-cultural communication. It was not child abuse.

My son David spent two years in Japan after college. He described the experience when he first arrived of feeling deaf, dumb, and illiterate—not speaking the language, not understanding the spoken language, and not able to read the language. The way Japanese write their numbers is unintelligible to us. They use Chinese numerals. Lia's parents may have been illiterate only with Arabic numbers. If the doctors caring for Lia had this knowledge, they might have done something as simple as marking the correct level on the tube with permanent ink or with tape.

My practice included occasional Hmong patients. I wish that I could tell you that I learned more about them. I learned a little, but it was very little. Once, when I saw a Hmong woman in the clinic, I took a chance that her culture might resemble Chinese culture, even though the Hmong left China generations ago because of their difficulties under the Chinese. With the woman were her teenage daughter, who spoke English and served as the translator, and her parents, who observed in silence. (These were the days before I had access to professional interpreters.)

At the end of the visit, I wrote out a prescription. I picked it up with both hands and passed it ceremoniously to the woman. This is considered good manners in China, where any piece of paper is passed as a valued document. I asked the girl who interpreted to ask her grandfather if he had any questions. The answer came back, "No." He shifted in his chair and smiled with pleasure. I had treated him with the respect due the oldest one in the room. I would like to think that my efforts at good Asian manners improved this intercultural interaction.

A third book to consider is Tracy Kidder's *Mountains Beyond Mountains*. It tells the story of Dr. Paul Farmer. Dr. Farmer's father was a free spirit, resulting in a chaotic childhood for Paul, much of it in Florida. One summer, the entire family worked alongside Haitian migrants harvesting citrus fruits. Later, Paul Farmer did exceptionally well at Duke University and Harvard Medical School. He continued his interest in the Haitians, traveling to their country and developing medical projects in Haiti's central plateau. With others he started Partners in Health, working in Haiti, Peru, and Russia. Dr. Farmer focused on high-quality, cost-effective care, including public health projects involving water supplies, sanitation systems, and vaccination programs.

There are other books that I have found helpful, but they are travel books I read for pleasure, with scattered insights into customs and history. If you want the pleasure, Paul Theroux's book *Plain of Snakes* is about Mexico. Colin Thubron's *Amur River* is about Mongolia, Russia, and China. An older book by Eric Newby, *A Short Walk in the Hindu Kush*, is about driving from London across Europe and parts of Asia to an adventure in Afghanistan.

There are many others, but this is a start. In our increasingly small and interconnected world, we need the education that travel provides. These authors permit travel while remaining in a favorite chair at home.

Latin America Culture

A colleague who worked in another hospital was hostile to Spanish-speaking patients. Speaking no Spanish himself, he communicated with the aid of an interpreter. He would ask each patient how long they had lived in this country. He would then criticize the patient for being here that long and not learning English. I heard about this second-hand, so I can only speculate that he sounds angry, perhaps at the delays involved when using an interpreter, or perhaps at himself for not having greater language skills.

Much earlier, before interpreters were required or even available, I had wanted to expand my private practice. The most underserved population in my community was Spanish-speaking. I purchased a recorded course called "Spanish I." I got no further than Spanish I, but it was enough to take most histories and communicate during physical examinations. To my surprise, some of the patients who had said that they did not speak English interrupted my Spanish to continue our conversation in English. Their flawed English was much better than my flawed Spanish.

A family practice resident from Panama explained this to me.

He said that every Spanish-speaking immigrant had been laughed at when they spoke English. When they heard my flawed Spanish, they knew that I would not ridicule their English.

My Spanish skills were sufficient so that I noticed their courtesies and good manners. Much later I read in a guidebook to Mexico that good manners are valued in Latin America more so than in the United States. I thought of the poor manners of my colleague who berated patients for not learning English. His critical attitude would have convinced his patients that they were right to hide their limited English.

In Central Massachusetts, where I practiced for many years, Spanish-speaking immigrants came primarily from Puerto Rico, but not exclusively. We also had a sizable group from Uruguay. They speak the same Spanish language but with a different accent and have a slightly different national culture. We had another sizable group from Brazil. They speak the closely related Portuguese language and have a third culture. Most of the Brazilian immigrants I met came from the flat interior agricultural states of Matto Grosso and Goias, in the regions around the capital, Brasilia. These areas have a different, more rural culture than the cities of Rio de Janeiro and Sao Paolo, just as rural cultures in the United States differ from urban cultures.

Imagine that you use a microscope with three magnifications to study a country's culture. At low magnification you see the country; at medium magnification you see a region within the country; and at high magnification you see the individual, who might be unexpectedly different from everyone else in the culture. Use only one of the three magnifications and you don't have the full picture.

In showing respect for the cultures of others, one need not forget one's own. I have had patients who came from corrupt countries who asked me to do things that I could not and would not do. They were testing and exploring limits. I needed to set good limits. Humanism includes an obligation to extend respect to others, but others have an obligation to respect us in return.

Arab Islamic Culture

An important culture that I know only a little about is the Arab Islamic culture. It has different rules from ours about touch and how much of the body can be exposed. I would urge young doctors to err on the side of caution before doing a physical examination on someone who observes Arab customs. Ask permission and explain what you are about to do.

A doctor from Lebanon told me that the customs of his people are lovely. I could see that he was comfortable in this country. He had learned our culture and our customs. He occasionally encountered bias against his background, which surprised him and was rude, but I observed that his good manners meant that he responded only with politeness. That response reflected well on his culture. As to our own culture, there have been changes during my lifetime, with generally increased humanity, but the progress has been uneven.

• • • • •

I will conclude this chapter with stories of three other cultures that I have encountered: the Scandinavian culture of Finland, the African culture of the Cameroons, and the south-Asian culture of the Bhutanese Nepalis. I offer these as illustrations of the rich variety of world cultures.

The American Finnish Community

There is a community of Finnish immigrants in the Mesabi Iron Range area of northern Minnesota. One of them, with the common Finnish last name of Maki, told me that until he went to school at the age of five or six, he thought that English was a foreign language. In his childhood he had the task of learning two cultures. There is another Finnish community in central Massachusetts where car signs read "SISU." A Finn told me "sisu" means "guts." Sisu is a stoical, stubborn determination that will see Finns through difficulties. From November 1939, to April 1940, during World War II, Russia attempted to occupy Finland in the Winter War. Finns fought on cross-country skis armed with hunting rifles, local knowledge, and sisu. That was sufficient for the Finns to achieve a stalemate against the more mechanized and more massive Russian army, maintaining their independence at that time.

A peace treaty ended the Winter War. It did not last long, for when Russia was attacked by Germany in 1941, Finland saw an opportunity to win back lost territory. Without going through all the details, with Russia victorious at the end of the war, Finland ceded 12 percent of its pre-war territory to its massive neighbor while maintaining its independence.

Finns tend to understate. A Finn who told me that he had a little discomfort might need relatively powerful hydrocodone or another mid-level narcotic to manage the pain of a fracture. He was proud of his sisu, and my task was to make it easy for him to be proud. Cultural norms can complicate communication about symptoms. Patients from other cultures would not say "a little discomfort" to describe the pain of a fracture. I needed to listen through a cultural filter.

The Cameroons

An immigrant from the Cameroons who had been in this country for years stubbed a toe on a curb in a parking lot, breaking her great toe. She was 60 years old, overweight, and had a problem with insurance since her health insurance carrier wanted the parking lot's insurance to cover her care. The insurance problems delayed her first visit with me until three weeks after the accident. The fracture had angulated her great toe so that it now pointed straight up. Had I seen it during the first day or two, I could have injected local anesthetic along nerves in the foot, straightened the toe, and taped it to the second toe, all easily done in the office. By three weeks after the accident it had healed sufficiently so that I needed anesthesia in the operating room to expose the fracture, refracture the bone using a chisel, straighten the deformity, and fix it with pins.

Then, to my dismay, the patient changed the dressing at home, pulling out the pins as she pulled off the old dressing. The patient had both generalized osteoporosis and local disuse osteoporosis in the toe that had developed during the delay in treatment. The pins had poor purchase in the softened bone. When the dressing pulled the pins out, the deformity recurred.

We returned to the operating room. I repeated the operation, this time putting on a unique cast that made it impossible for the pins to back out and, in addition, made it impossible for anyone without a cast saw to change the dressing.

The patient announced that she could not return for the follow-up visit that I recommended. She was returning to the Cameroons for a visit. She would see me when she returned. I wanted her to delay the trip until the fracture had healed, the pins were out, and the cast was off. If she went to Africa with the cast and the pins, I worried about her walking long distances in the heat and dust on dirt roads in poorly-developed areas. She could have a complicating infection involving the pins with no access to modern medical care.

She made an informed decision to ignore my advice.

When she did return to see me after her return from the Cameroons, I removed the cast and the pins. To my great relief, the fracture had healed, the toe was straight, and no infection had occurred. I removed the pins in the office, and except for one more follow-up visit as a precaution, the treatment was complete.

I asked about her pressing need to return to the Cameroons. She explained that she had been ignoring the earth. The earth is our mother. It provides us with food. We return to our mother when we die. With the trouble with her toe, she went back to the Cameroons to rectify her neglect of the earth. She paid a large amount of money to two priests who spent 24 hours with her in a ceremony of atonement. After that her toe had healed. The priests had been critical of her turning to me for treatment. She had defended me to them, for she now was a woman of two cultures.

Even though I eventually achieved an excellent result in this case, I can't be proud of my care. I can't be proud of our medical system. With our system delaying needed care and with my needing two trips to the operating room, I was not surprised that she fell back on the beliefs of her childhood. Our care had not done enough to inspire sufficient confidence.

I have tried to imagine what it is like for an immigrant to grow old in this country, with decreasing mentation and increasing health problems. Our health care system may be very different from what the immigrant trusted as a child, as it was in this case. The responsibility, respect, and empathy that define humane medical care mean being sensitive to trust issues.

The Bhutanese Nepalis

The last case that I will discuss involves a Bhutanese Nepali. I had to look up their story on Wikipedia. Early in the 20th century, a group of Nepalis had moved to Bhutan, another small country bordering India, to work as farmers and carpenters or other tradespeople. They were industrious and did well. Their success led to Bhutanese resentment, so that the Bhutanese then discriminated against them. Organizers persuaded the Nepali immigrants to stand up for their rights. Some of them did. The Bhutanese responded by expelling those agitating for their rights and, along with them, all the rest of the Bhutanese Nepalis. Nepal, a poor country on which they had once turned their backs, refused to accept their return.

Homeless and destitute, many Bhutanese Nepali went to camps in India and from there to this country. Some of them settled in central Massachusetts. I would see Bhutanese Nepali patients from time to time, using the service of our single Nepalese interpreter. This interpreter had been a Nepali mathematics teacher in Bhutan. Occasionally I joined him in the cafeteria for lunch, finding him alone, eating quietly while reading the Nepalese poetry he loved.

He taught me to greet his people respectfully with the Buddhist word "Namaste." His pay as an interpreter was low. He attended night school to qualify for the better job of a social worker and to continue to serve his people from that position.

One of the patients whom I saw with him was a man of about 50 with back pain that did not come from his back but came instead from an old fracture of his left femur, just below the hip, in the subtrochanteric region. The fracture had healed with shortening and with angulation of 80 degrees. To stand or walk, he had to compensate for the deformity of his thigh by twisting his back. The treatment for this would be done in our fracture clinic by an operation on the malunion of the femur and not in the spine clinic where I saw him. The fracture surgeons would cut through the bone at the deformity, correct the deformity, and secure the two parts of the bone in the corrected position with a rod and screws or another fixation device. Recovery would be rapid, with a short stay in the hospital until he could walk independently on crutches and perhaps three months until he healed well enough to discard the crutches.

He did not go to the fracture clinic, but he did return to see me a second and third time. The third time was during a snowstorm that had resulted in cancellations of many visits. That allowed me to spend more time with him. Through the interpreter, I asked why he had not gone to the fracture clinic. He avoided answering. I asked if he was afraid of amputation or death, knowing that these were common and feared outcomes of hospital stays in the third world. He said no. I assured him that neither would happen, leaving out the usual qualification, "unlikely to happen." A long discussion in Nepalese followed between the patient and the interpreter. The interpreter then told me that the patient was concerned about feces, using the four-letter vulgarity for feces that I had never heard him use before.

The interpreter told me that when the patient first came to this country, he had lived in California. He worked for cash, under-the-table and without legal protections, for a tree service. A fall from a tree caused his fracture. He had no health insurance. His employer had no insurance. The patient could not get health care in the hospital. For a year, he lay in a bed. No one cleaned him so that he lay in his feces. The fracture healed, and he was able to get up again. He dreaded a recurrence of that convalescence and the filth he had endured.

I assured him that if he had the surgery, he would be able to get up on crutches immediately afterward, in the recovery room if necessary, and go to the bathroom. His face brightened. He agreed that he would do it.

This would be a better story if he had followed through. He never went to the fracture clinic, and never had the corrective surgery. I had tried to understand his concerns. I thought that he had changed his mind. He may have, but if he did, he changed it back again later.

The bad result of his treatment in California suggests a failure of our health care system. Be careful. Justice, one of the four pillars of ethical medicine, requires hearing both sides of a story before judging. It is possible this man refused care in California. If he did, it could have involved the same mistrust of Western medicine that I encountered and never overcame.

I had learned bits and pieces about the interpreter's life. Through no fault of his own, this good man lost a respected position in Bhutan. After a time in a camp in India, he came to this country. He had the energy to begin his economic and social recovery, but not to the level he had in Bhutan. He was perhaps 30 years old, unmarried, but young enough to start a new career, and, if he chose to do so, to marry and have a family. As the immigrant generation, his life will never be as good as it would have been had things turned out differently in Bhutan. It will be the next generation—his children if he has any—who will prosper.

That pattern is repeated with each wave of immigrants. Many decide to come here only after things become desperate at home. Giving up community roots can be hard; most do it only under great duress. Many fail to return to the social and economic levels that they knew before they were forced to move. The members of the second generation may be the ones who experience the social and economic benefits of the move.

• • • • •

This concludes our discussion of cultures. While I have been able to travel widely and to unusual places, some of my greatest cultural encounters have been here in central Massachusetts. I needed to travel no further than from one examining room to the next. These encounters have been among the great privileges and great pleasures of being a doctor. I suggest that you be open, curious, respectful, and empathetic with immigrants. You will be rewarded with your own memorable experiences.

Next we turn to challenging situations encountered in medical practice.

Chapter Ten

Challenging Clinical Situations

This chapter considers challenging clinical situations that may occur in any medical specialty that includes interactions with patients. Others before us have thought about these situations and techniques to manage them. One of the techniques is transactional analysis, which I will introduce next, followed by seven clinical challenges for you to think about now, when you have the time, before your encounters with them later, when you may not have time to think.

Transactional Analysis

Eric Berne, M.D., a psychiatrist, developed transactional analysis. He described it in *Games People Play* and other publications. When two people interact, each can assume one of three roles. One is the Parent ego state, or more simply the Parent, one is the Adult, and one is the Child. The Parent uses the verbs "ought" or "should" and is concerned with values, ethics, and caring. The Adult uses the verb "can" and is concerned with problem-solving and logic. The Child uses the verbs "want," "love," "hate," and "fear" and is concerned with the emotions of childhood, including positive joy and negative hate and fear. The Child has a sense of playfulness.

These three ego states are similar to Freud's superego, ego, and id, except that Freud's terms apply to the mental processes within an individual, and the transactional terms apply to external relationships. Berne's Parent involves caring in addition to the judging that the superego does. Berne's Child involves charm, creativity, and playfulness that are not part of the id and perhaps less sexuality than the id.

Berne describes what he has named a simple transaction between two people. For instance, a patient says, "I have pain in my stomach when I eat spicy food and drink beer." The doctor says, "That could be an ulcer. We will need to order tests."

The patient and the doctor are logical and seek to solve a problem. This is Berne's simple transaction. Both parties accept an Adult-Adult social transaction. There is no hidden psychological transaction and no ulterior motive. There can be other simple transactions, with common types being Parent-Child and Child-Child.

An interaction may be crossed. The patient says, "I have pain in my stomach." The doctor responds, "You should stop drinking with your rowdy friends."

The patient has initiated what might be an Adult-Adult interaction, while the doctor has initiated what might be a Parent-Child interaction. The two are working at cross-purposes. Berne has a way of diagramming interactions. The line from patient's Adult on the left to the doctor's Adult on the right crosses the line back from the doctor's Parent on the right to the patient's Child on the left.

Berne says that crossed interactions soon end. When I have seen crossed interactions that did not end quickly, it was generally because one of the participants had an ulterior motive. Berne would consider that a game, which we will get to, but first we will consider complex interactions.

Complex transactions involve a social transaction, which is more obvious, and a psychological transaction, which may be hidden. The social transaction can be the Adult in the patient saying I have pain, and the Adult in the doctor saying, I will order tests.

The psychological transaction can be the Child in the patient expressing worry, perhaps with tone and body language only, and the Parent in the doctor saying, don't worry, I will take care of this, again perhaps also with tone and body language only.

A game is a transaction with a concealed ulterior motive to obtain a payoff. It is the manipulative concealment plus the payoff that makes this a game, even if part or all is subconscious or hidden from one or both parties.

As an example, I once had a patient with Dupuytren's contracture, or progressive fibrosis and contracture of the fascia just beneath the skin on the palm of the hands. It can be painful and cause deformities. As the disease progressed and new areas of fibrosis developed, this patient repeatedly asked me to operate. This appeared to be an Adult-Adult transaction. Still, I was operating about every six months for relatively minor pathology.

The patient was a poor soul, skinny, impoverished, and isolated. He worked at menial tasks for a distant relative who knew his limited talents and had taken pity on him. A great pleasure that the patient described to me was a fish he had caught in a local stream and made into one of his best meals. The game we were playing involved a social Adult-Adult transaction, with the patient requesting surgery and my providing it. The hidden psychological transaction was Child-Parent, with the patient's Child receiving caring attention from my Parent and from the caring staff in my office. The concealed payoff was the patient's feeling while getting medical attention. It was a feeling that he rarely had outside of his medical visits. It may have been the feeling of being valued and cared for.

On the advice of two psychiatrist friends, I started seeing the patient in my office every three months, ostensibly to check on the contracture. My friends, the psychiatrists, saw that the surgery would not be necessary if the patient received our office's attention without it. They were correct. With his visits to us every three months he never again asked for surgery.

Eric Berne was, and I believe still is, a controversial figure within psychiatry. He was a licensed physician who successfully completed psychiatric residency but was denied admission to the San Francisco Psychoanalytic Institute, perhaps because his ideas were unconventional. Studies have shown that his system can be used effectively. One of my colleagues used it in a program directed at smoking cessation. Another does not use it but emphasizes relationships between individuals in her practice, using other theories that have developed in the decades since Freud's brilliant and pioneering work focused on individuals, neglecting relationships.

• • • • •

Let us now turn to the central subject of this chapter—challenging situations. These challenging situations can be upsetting, but that is rare, and most of your encounters with patients will be less upsetting, so don't let this catalogue of troubles worry you. Take comfort in knowing that, as you gain experience and develop your skills, the upsetting challenges will become increasingly rare.

Dealing With Tragedy

One challenging situation is dealing with tragedy. I recently heard from a medical student who is part of Budd Shenkin's humanistic medicine initiative. She had listened to a discussion of a woman in her 20s whose brain tumor continued growing despite surgery, despite everything the oncologists could do, and despite everything that the radiotherapists could offer. The discussion was comprehensive and scholarly in the best medical school tradition and, respecting another, more questionable tradition, without emotion.

The student said that it was only while walking home afterward that it occurred to her: "A woman my age is going to die, and there is nothing that we can do for her. That is awful!"

This is an example of the tragedy that we as doctors encounter repeatedly and the way that we may isolate ourselves from our feelings or repress them. Freud described these two processes as defense mechanisms. Kuebler Ross regarded denial as the first stage in grief, using "denial" rather than "isolation" or "repression." Often it is necessary to isolate, repress, or deny our feelings while dealing with a case, or even for hours afterward, until our shift is over. Having the feelings while walking home is healthy. Never admitting to the feelings is not. The danger is that our feelings are simmering in the subconscious, building up pressure that will explode and cause us trouble later.

During training, we frequently need to protect ourselves from feeling the full tragedy of the worst cases. Pain and suffering after surgery? Buck up, we think of telling the patient, that is expected and a small price for them to pay for essential surgery. Breaking ribs massaging the heart during cardiopulmonary resuscitation? Forget the ribs and focus on saving a life. The young man screaming in pain after a multi-car accident? Ignore him and focus on the older, deathly pale patient in the same car wreck who is only softly moaning. That is the patient who will die without immediate attention. We experience tragedy, learn technical skills, protect ourselves from intense emotions, and teach ourselves to be cold and uncaring.

Don't be surprised if those ahead of you, including residents and fellows, appear unfeeling. It is their defense against intense and even paralyzing emotions. Unfortunately, callousness is not humanistic. It is not respectful. It blocks empathy. Hopefully, those who have become callous in training will recover a more humanistic approach later.

One of Freud's great insights was that psychological defenses are not perfect. The isolated emotion does not remain isolated, the repressed emotion doesn't remain repressed, and the denied emotion can make a later surprise and disruptive reappearance.

Most of us in my generation managed without psychiatric help, but sometimes at the price of leaving clinical medicine altogether. That is not the best role model for you young doctors. Please seek help when you are distressed. You might begin by talking to a trusted friend.

Giving Bad News

A second challenging situation is giving bad news. One of the hardest things that we must do is to tell a patient that they have cancer. That happens less often in orthopaedics than in some other specialties, so that my own experience is limited. What follows is what I was taught.

First, as the results of tests come back, the patient may ask for the results. When they ask, they are ready to hear the news. Before they ask, their denial may be so strong that they will not remember what you say.

Second, spend the time needed with the patient after telling them the news. This time may be an hour. Don't waste time by talking all around the issue and avoiding the word "cancer." That suggests anxieties on your part, which is your problem, not the patient's. Your discomfort can only increase the patient's. Come right out and say "cancer" early. Then be with the patient to offer sympathy. Answer questions honestly. If there is hope of successful treatment, offer it, but do not offer false hope. False hope destroys the trust that you and the patient will need later.

Just once a patient asked me what the diagnosis was when I simply could not devote the time needed after giving bad news. I had another patient whose problems were even more pressing. In that case, I was able to ask a physician's assistant to step in and offer the support that I should have given the patient but could not provide.

Third, if the patient doesn't ask and too much time goes by, bring up the subject yourself. Family members may ask you not to tell a parent, saying that the parent is not strong and couldn't take the shock. That is wrong. The patient knows that something is not right. He/she becomes increasingly isolated because no one will discuss what is wrong. It is more caring and more supportive to include the patient. The request from the family member suggests that the family member is having problems with the news. You may need to spend time with that family member.

Fourth and finally, once having told the patient, don't bring up the subject again unnecessarily. There is no need to tell the patient on every visit that what they have is terrible. That suggests you are having a problem with the situation and want to distance yourself. Just be honest, be open, and be humane.

In orthopaedics, the bad news that I had for patients was more likely a chronic disease or a permanent disability. The most common chronic disease was osteoarthritis. The most serious permanent disability was paralysis after a spine fracture. While the news of a chronic disease or permanent disability may not be as severe as the news of impending death, the patients were often younger. The older patients were more accepting of bad news. The guidelines for informing patients about cancer can be useful with any bad news.

Perhaps the mildest bad news that I had for patients was that they needed to restrict their activities for a time to allow a fracture to heal. This amounts to a significant but temporary disability in return for a life afterward of full recovery. Patients would respond, "What do you mean, not work? I have a business to run and a family to support." Or, "What do you mean, rest? My daughter is getting married this weekend, and I have to walk her down the aisle." Or, "What do you mean, not drive? The cast is on my right foot. I can drive with my left."

All of these responses are forms of denial. For you to gain adherence to a good treatment plan, you must address denial. Failure to address denial can lead to treatment failure and permanent consequences. Take responsibility, be beneficent, and address it. Address it with respect and empathy, but address it.

I will conclude this section by acknowledging that my experiences are already dated. The 2016 U. S. 21st Century Cures Act is now on the books. The main portions of the act simplify or weaken the processes that industries use to get approvals for new treatments. One small portion of the act gives patients full and unrestricted access to their medical records. Failure of an institution to comply can result in a fine of $1 million. Because of this Act, now it may not be the doctor who gives the patient bad news and then offers emotional support. The patient may get the bad news from a screen anywhere with access to the internet—a coffee shop, perhaps—and may get it with no access to emotional support. This is an increase in transparency that will have unforeseen consequences. One of the challenges today and in the near future for the medical community will be how we might help in dealing with these consequences.

The Patient You Do Not Like

A third challenging clinical situation is treating a patient whom you do not like. One version of this is that you do not know the patient, but he or she is a member of a group that is opposed to your group. You are a Palestinian doctor, and a wounded Israeli soldier is brought to you, or you are a Catalan doctor and an injured Madrid politician is brought to you.

My physician father and I discussed this subject when I was an intern. I was caring for a 19-year-old woman who had been an unrestrained front-seat passenger in a car accident. It was 1967, before air bags and when only a few cars had seat belts. She was unconscious in Intensive Care and had bilateral severe lung contusions. I felt awful that she should be the severely injured victim of such a tragedy. I said something like what Dr. Francis Peabody had said, that because I cared about what had happened to this patient I was working extra hard. My father disagreed. He said you work hard for every patient because of your professional pride. Otherwise, what happens when you have a patient that you don't like?

Later in my career I had patients that I didn't like. Following my father's advice, I worked hard because of my professional pride. Surprisingly often, as days went by, I began to like the patient. Empathy followed. What started as working because of pride became working because of caring.

Empathy does not always come. I had, as you will have, troubled relationships with patients. In a relationship, there is you, me, and us—there is the patient, there is the doctor, and there is the relationship. The approach to a troubled relationship depends on which part is troubled.

If it is the patient, it may help to ask yourself, "What is the opposite?" We have considered this before. The opposite of the angry patient may be a frightened patient. The opposite of an imposing or arrogant patient may be one who feels inferior. If you can deal with the fear or the insecurity, your relationship may improve.

Another problem is the double bind. That is when the patient makes two demands, but meeting one makes it impossible to meet the other. A patient can demand the doctor treat a heart problem but with natural remedies only. Prescription medications are unacceptable.

As an orthopaedic surgeon, my exposure to double binds was mainly with Jehovah's Witnesses who refused blood transfusions. I felt that in urgent or emergency situations, I would operate with that restriction but that in elective situations, I would not do surgery. The patient was welcome to seek care from another doctor who might have different ethics from mine. The law is that a doctor-patient relationship is voluntary on both sides, so long as there is time for the patient to find another doctor. In an emergency, I would not abandon the patient, and I could not by law. In an elective situation, I could follow my own understanding of beneficence and non-maleficence. I had that right.

When a patient wants to limit care, consider having a discussion to learn more about the patient's reasons and to explain your own reasons. That might be followed by negotiation, trying to find a compromise that would satisfy both of you. If you can't find a compromise, consider withdrawing from the case, but only at a future date that gives the patient time to find another doctor.

A special case of the patient whom you don't like is an abusive or threatening patient. My teaching was to set limits with the abusive patient and call for help with the threatening patient. Patients have rights and also responsibilities, one of which is not to abuse. Medical personnel have responsibilities and also rights, one of which is not to be abused. I have told patients who mistreated the receptionist that the mistreatment was unacceptable. My plan was that, with a second occurrence of mistreatment, I would warn the patient of possible discharge from the practice, and with a third occurrence of abuse, I would discharge the patient. As it turned out, the first warning was always enough.

With a threatening patient, I have had little experience. I am a big guy, so an average-sized patient would hesitate to threaten me. I have been in examining rooms with other big guys whose anger was increasing. I found ways to leave the room, and in one case, the staff and I agreed to call the police.

The most frightened I have been was in a situation outside medicine. At a public gathering well outside my neighborhood (if a prairie in South Dakota south of the Badlands can be considered a neighborhood), a dozen men surrounded me and wanted money. My fear reminded me of the fear that I have felt when large dogs turned aggressive. With the dogs, it was important that I act neither like predator nor prey. With the dogs, I would speak calmly, not aggressively, and move slowly and obliquely away, rather than running directly away like prey. With the men who surrounded me, I did something like this: I declined the request, stood quietly, not moving (I was surrounded), and asked by name whether two people whom I knew who lived in the area had come to the gathering. It turned out that the men who had surrounded me were, like me, not from the area. One of the people I mentioned was from a locally prominent family. My connections may have frightened them, for they dispersed.

Perhaps something in this story will help you some day.

Let us turn to the doctor's side of the relationship. A doctor can experience cognitive dissonance. Two of the three parts of this condition are in the name. The doctor has cognition, or recognition, of something that is dissonant, or clashes with the third part, a belief or habit. (The third part is left out of the name, cognitive dissonance. A more complete description of the condition is (1) the cognition of something that is (2) dissonant with (3) a current belief or habit from the past.

Imagine that you are on a clinical rotation and have been up all night with a complex and very sick patient who is finally getting better. You did an exceptional job keeping the patient alive. You stumble exhaustedly into morning rounds. The attending finds out that you do not know the radiologist's reading of the chest X-ray that has just appeared on the computer. The attending says, "You didn't finish your work, did you?"

What you feel—a mixture of disappointment, confusion, abandonment, and anger—is cognitive dissonance. The cognition is of the attending's criticism. The dissonance is with what you know to have been exceptional patient care.

Be careful of anger. Automobile race car drivers refer to "the red mist of rage." Even before you get to that level, anger is an excellent indication to walk away and calm down. There is an aphorism, "Act in haste, repent at leisure." Don't act too hastily.

In addition to problems centered on the patient and those centered on the doctor, there are problems that center on the relationship. One relationship problem involves the scripts for the medical visit. Your script may be to work from the chief complaint toward a diagnosis and a treatment plan. If the patient gives a chief complaint that is not the real problem, you probably have conflicting scripts. The clue to the conflicting scripts may be the patient's urge to talk about matters extraneous to the chief complaint.

Conflicting scripts may involve Berne's crossed transactions, but not necessarily. Patient and doctor may agree on a simple Adult-Adult transaction and still have different goals in the transaction.

If patient and doctor do not agree on a transaction type, then they have a problem with their relationship. The doctor may have addressed the patient's Child, and the patient wants the Adult recognized. Or the doctor may have assumed the Parent role and preached, while the patient only wants the logical explanations of the doctor's Adult. When my son-in-law was asked on an initial visit with a medical practioner, "What do you think we should do?" he was upset. That question sounded like a question from a Child to a Parent. My son-in-law was looking for an Adult or a Parent who could help him.

Sex Between a Doctor and Patient

A fourth challenging situation involves sex between a doctor and a patient. This is the problem of the patient you like, and you like them because you find them sexually attractive. We will explore the you-me-us aspects of this, but first, let me say, "NO!"

The rule is this: no sex with a patient. There should be no exceptions. As doctors, we are responsible for the health of our patients. We need to inspect and palpate any part of the body, including the most private parts, for the private parts also develop diseases. That privilege is allowed us with the understanding that we will use it responsibly and only for professional reasons. If a doctor violates that understanding, it threatens the public's trust in all of us. A lack of trust in doctors becomes a threat to everyone's health. Your hospital understands that, your state board of medical licensure understands that, and the court system understands that. Failure to control your sex drive means trouble. That trouble could destroy your career.

To explore this topic further, when sexual feelings enter the doctor-patient relationship, consider you, me, and us—that is, you, the patient; or me, the doctor; or us, our doctor-patient relationship. We will begin with you, the patient.

A patient may be seductive. Why? The most innocent reason would be the magical thinking that a special relationship with the doctor might be the best way to obtain a cure. A second reason for a patient to be seductive was illustrated by a friend who was blackmailed by two women who claimed he behaved indecently. A third reason would be sexual arousal in the patient independent of anything that the doctor did. Don't flatter yourself. That is a rare reason for a patient to behave seductively.

Or it is possible that it is us—the relationship—that got derailed. Do not participate in flirtatious banter. The first rule is no sex. Does sex include flirtatious banter? It is close enough, so don't. It is too dangerous.

The third possibility is me, the doctor. If you feel sexual arousal, admit it to yourself. It doesn't matter if it might have been provoked. Your arousal is a possibility that creates fear and even terror in patients who already feel vulnerable. Make sure that there is a third person in the room during the visit, even while taking the history. Don't examine breasts, genital organs, or rectum. If you experience arousal, you probably should transfer the patient to another doctor so that this will be your last visit with this patient.

Borderline Patients

A fifth challenging situation is the patient with a borderline personality disorder. In the chapter on psychiatry, we discussed this diagnosis. Suspect it if your relationship with the patient is volatile. During one visit you are a glorious hero up on a pedestal, and during the next visit you are a despicable bum down in the gutter. You don't know what you might have done to cause this volatility. You feel like you are walking on eggshells and you can't walk carefully enough.

Borderline patients are very difficult, even for psychiatrists. These patients may complain if you are empathetic. Their complaint won't be about the empathy; it will be about something else, but it is the empathy that feels engulfing and overwhelming to the patient. They will also complain if you are too distant. Again, the complaint will be about something else, but it is the distance that feels like abandonment that is the problem. The eggshells that break belong to the patient.

In any challenging case, remember that you are not alone. The hospital will have resources. With a borderline patient, consider a psychiatry consult. In other challenging cases, think about calling in a social worker, chaplain, legal counsel, or patient representative or ombudsperson from the office that deals with medical care complaints.

For you young doctors, up until now, you have never been allowed to whisper to your neighbor during school tests. Now, as you enter medical practice, you are expected to talk to another physician when you are tested by a clinical situation and you are uncertain. This can be a new experience for you. When it is the best thing to do, assemble a team to address a complex problem.

The Screaming Toddler

A sixth challenging situation is the screaming toddler. At its worst, the situation includes a screaming child, an angry parent, and a frustrated doctor. Remember, the child understands little of your words and less of your logic but everything about your tone and body language. Be careful about looming over the child or cornering the child. Stay calm and non-threatening. You can be as firm as necessary but never in anger. Respect the child's need to gain trust in you, the doctor. That takes time, but you may save time later when everything else becomes easier. Pay attention to the parent-child relationships. The child depends on the parents for love and protection, and now they are worried and confused. There is this third relationship in the room, in addition to your relationship with the child and your relationship with the parents. This third relationship doesn't involve you, except that it does.

Children are even more sensitive to inhumanity than adults. Be careful and gentle with them.

Long-Term and Public Health Concerns

A seventh challenge involves extending yourself beyond the more obvious acute care that is needed now by your patient and thinking about your patient long-term and the community. This challenge differs from specialty to specialty. Primary caregivers already think more about the long-term, while orthopaedic surgeons may think about it less and may focus more on *this* problem in *this* patient at *this* moment.

At some point in my practice, I realized that I was seeing repeat fractures. One pattern of a repeated fracture was the older woman with a previous hip fracture who returned with the other hip fractured. I began to do osteoporosis studies on every patient with a hip fracture. About a quarter had either low levels of Vitamin D or secondary hyperparathyroidism, usually due to renal disease. Both conditions can be treated. The treatment does not reverse their osteoporosis, but it does stop the downward trend of the untreated disease. I set myself the goal of treating this fracture and preventing the next one. It is easy for an orthopaedic surgeon to say, "Osteoporosis is not my responsibility." That is true in theory, but in practice the tests weren't happening unless I ordered them. Shrugging off the responsibility would not be responsible and could be maleficent. Ordering them was beneficent.

Another pattern of repeated fractures was the pre-adolescent boy with wild ways. I began to give a speech to any boy with a second fracture. I made a comic reference to a metaphoric yellow caution light that goes on in the back of the head indicating danger and excitement. The boy with repeated fractures had been ignoring the danger and enjoying the excitement. I would not be there the next time the yellow caution light goes on, nor would his parents. It was up to him to choose between danger and excitement. If he chose excitement again, he was likely to end up in my office again, for another cast and the weeks of treatment that would follow.

Once I started giving this speech, I never saw a third fracture. There may have been third fractures that were treated by others. Still, I wasn't seeing them in the way that I had, which is an indication that I was doing better at treating this fracture and preventing the next one.

A different case of thinking more broadly began on a Sunday after a Saturday snowstorm. Sunday was bright and warm, so that the snow that had fallen all through the night was now moist and heavy. This heavy, moist snow clogged the exit chutes of the snow blowers that homeowners used to clear their sidewalks and driveways. People were reaching into their snow blowers to remove the clogged snow. One patient after another came into the emergency room with fingertip amputations, usually close to the last joint, just before or just after the distal interphalangeal joint. Even when the operator of the snow blower has turned it off, there could be tension in the engine or the drive that caused the impeller to move far enough once the clog was cleared to amputate fingertips.

The surgical challenge is to retain as much length as possible while still closing the amputation with viable, innervated skin that is thick enough to stand up to heavy use. Often this involves moving a local, V-shaped flap of skin distally to cover exposed bone. That Sunday I took nine patients to the operating room to close amputations. The anesthesiologist grumbled, "You have to tell people not to stick their hands into their snow blowers."

On Monday I found the administrator who dealt with the hospital's public relations. He was non-committal about getting the word out. Nothing happened on the next two days, and I had almost forgotten about the matter when, on Thursday, an article appeared in our local paper. On Friday, the health reporter for a Boston TV station and her videographer drove the hour from Boston to interview me. She suggested that we go to the Emergency Department where she interviewed me standing next to the x-ray view box that we used then. On the view box we placed an x-ray image of a hand with an amputated fingertip. A videographer filmed the interview. Afterwards she told me that this was already old news, so that they would save the interview and broadcast it when the next snowstorm occurred.

Several weeks later the station broadcast the interview. I looked stiff and camera-shy, but that was not the point. The point was to save at least a few fingertips. We may have done that, not only in the area around our own community but also in the wider Boston metropolitan area.

My father was the health officer in the small town where I grew up. While I was in high school, he became involved in adding fluoride to the water supply. A few members of the community were vocal in their opposition to this measure. While I was in college he organized a study involving all of the local dentists and a researcher from the University of Wisconsin Medical School in Madison. It compared the number of cavities filled in children before and after the introduction of fluoride. Fluoridation led to a significant decrease in cavities. He never told me about the study. I don't think that it was ever published. I think that he needed it for sessions of the City Council that responded to ongoing complaints about fluoridation. I first learned about the study after he had died. I was clearing out his possessions when I found a copy of the report saved among other treasured family documents.

I believe that my father took pleasure in the effort that went into this public health study, just as I took pleasure in the public health efforts that I have made. For both of us, medicine was more than making a living; it was a calling. At times we did more than the minimum because that is what you do when your work is not a nine-to-five job tolerated only because of the paycheck. Neither of us burned out. My father worked until age 79 before retiring, and I worked until age 78. Both of us continued with volunteer medical activities after retiring.

For you who are starting out, it is your values, your humanism, and your ethics that will make the difference between medicine as only a job and medicine as a calling. It will be harder for you than it was for us because of increased reasons for burnout today. Your employers may treat you as if your work is only a job and not the calling with the ideals that you have learned. If you can, find a place where you can live up to your own ideals, even if it means a lower income. I wish you well. It may not be easy.

• • • • •

In the next chapter and the last one before the conclusion, we will consider five roles that a physician may fill during a lifetime in medicine.

Chapter Eleven

Five Medical Roles

In this chapter, we will consider the role of student and four other roles that you may choose to fill during your medical career. These are the roles of clinician, teacher, researcher, and administrator. A medical school education prepares you primarily for the role of clinician. Should you choose one of the other roles, you may need to devote extra time to studying education, research, or administration.

The Role of Student

For those now in medical school, please use this time well. That is your ethical responsibility. At the same time, don't overburden yourself. Set aside time for recreation. It is not all about tomorrow. Enjoy today as well. You may have already established this balance. It is a balance that you will need throughout life. This balance can sustain your energy for your main responsibility now as a student, which is preparing for your future responsibilities. Your job of preparing will be easier if you emphasize most what you need to do next. If you don't have the time to learn everything that you might want, emphasize what you will need in the next few years. As a medical student, emphasize preparation for your first post-graduate year. In the junior years of your post-graduate training, emphasize preparation for your senior years.

You will have electives. You can choose them because they interest you, or because they might be useful to you later, or because other students found them well-taught. One of my errors in choosing electives involved a poorly taught course that should have been useful but what little I learned I taught myself. One of my successes was a course I thought would be interesting but of little use in my own career. It was pediatric cardiology, where I learned to recognize the different heart murmurs with a stethoscope. That proved to be a very useful skill in my seemingly unrelated field of orthopaedics. It meant that I found damaged heart valves in my patients preoperatively and could seek appropriate consultations early.

If you find yourself in a course that is badly taught, make the most of it. Badly taught is not the same as poorly learned. You may have had this experience already. Even poor teachers will teach you a little. At a minimum, they are negative examples from which you can learn. You learn not just from the teacher but also from the experience, from other students, from nurses and physicians' assistants and other health care workers, and from books, articles, and on-line sites. Do not assume that you can learn only from the professors. They may be the furthest from the basic skills you need to master. Take advantage of the entire community around you in medical school. Everyone can help you.

As a student, you may experience the imposter syndrome. Pauline Clance and Suzanne Innes first identified this syndrome in women in 1978. Since then it has been recognized equally frequently in men. If you experience the imposter syndrome, you may think your school has made a mistake, that you do not deserve to be in medical school, and that you are an imposter. This may be a form of cognitive dissonance—the dissonance between what you have thought about yourself and what you think a medical degree will mean. The role you will play as a medical doctor will be different from any that you have played before, but that would be true whatever career you might choose. The imposter syndrome occurs to young people in every field. I have worked on various admissions committees. I know the quality of the applicants, including those whom we turned down. No, the school didn't make a mistake when it admitted you. What I know, and what those who admitted you know, is that you are capable of being a doctor—not an imposter, but a real doctor. Your professional personality will become a combination of the personalities of other doctors you have observed, what your position in medicine demands, and what unique characteristics you bring to your career. You will grow into being a doctor. You will be great.

You will need to decide on a specialty. In choosing, consider Freud's superego, ego, and id. The superego deals with values. Do something that you believe has value. You may want to consider what your archetype of a good doctor is. My archetype was a clinician, so pure research or pure administration wouldn't have satisfied me. Paul Farmer's archetype, or at least his values, included serving Haitians, which led him to his unique career.

The ego deals with practical matters. Do something for which you have talents and abilities. My talents lay more in physics than chemistry, so that orthopaedics was a good fit for me. You may want to consider the income that you will make, where you might live, and work-life balance. As for income, you will have enough to live well at some modest salary. Increments above that level make less and less difference to your quality of life. Do consider that a medical career can squeeze one's finances because of student debts at the beginning and fewer productive years to save for retirement at the end. Where you might live includes in a city, in a small town, or in the country near mountains, lakes, or an ocean. If you have chosen a high degree of specialization, there may be fewer centers where you might work. Consider your established networks of relatives and friends for your family and professional contacts for you. You may consider moving to a new section of the country, which would mean establishing new networks.

The id deals with feelings. A good specialty for you is one where you enjoy the work. You won't enjoy everything every day. That's life. But there should be some things about your specialty that gives you pleasure during some of the days.

The id deals with negative feelings as well as positive ones. Each specialty has its burden of negatives. The burdens in some specialties will be more acceptable to you than the burdens in others. One of my colleagues, who specialized in ear, nose, and throat surgery, found the odor of feet offensive. He did not understand how I could do orthopaedics. For me, the odor of feet was entirely acceptable and not a negative at all.

The Transition after Training

When your training is complete, you will need to find a job. The decision about your first job is a major and complex life decision. There are many factors to consider. Some factors are quantitative and can be measured and some are qualitative. An example of a measurable factor is income. An example of a qualitative factor is prestige. Don't be dazzled by either to the point that you are blinded to other important factors.

You will want to consider income but be careful with the offer of the highest income. The job with the best income may be at an extreme. An extreme that is desirable may be balanced by other extremes that are undesirable. The job with an extreme income may also have extremely long hours, extremely short times to spend with each patient, and extreme pressure to over-work. There is a saying that better is the enemy of good. In this case, the better salary may be enemy of good working conditions. Be careful.

You will also want to consider prestige, but the job at the most prestigious institution is also an extreme. It may be the best job for you, but, as you already know, there are unhappy people at the best institutions. There are also happy people there, so don't rule out a job because of prestige, but evaluate the position as carefully as you would a less prestigious one.

Include your significant other in any decision. Both of you will need to be happy with your decision, or neither of you will be happy.

While the decision is complex, don't make it too complex. No position will be perfect. Buddhists teach that you can never perfectly satisfy your wants, but you can perfectly not want. Suppose that the job is perfect except that your office will have no windows. Can you perfectly not want windows? You probably can.

When considering a position, chat with the secretaries or administrators during your visits. Have there been frequent turnovers of personnel? If there have, those in charge may mistreat underlings. You will start as an underling.

Try to sense the ethos of the organization. If the organization's ethos is one of money and social status and yours is one of service and scholarship, you probably won't be happy there.

You may want to ask yourself how easy or difficult you might find the job in the first year, and also where you might be in five or ten years. Is there a market for the services you have to offer in the community that you are considering? Those who offer you a position may have thoughts about this. Since they may be reluctant to talk about negatives, you may also want to ask for advice from those who have trained you and to ask those a few years ahead of you about their experiences.

It is easy to make a hurried decision about your future during the intensity of your final months in training. The time saved on a hasty decision may cost a great deal of time later in correcting the error. Take time with that first decision. Get advice. Talk it over with those whom you trust. Put in whatever effort is needed.

Once you are in the first position, do what you can to make it work. It won't be perfect. Every position has its drawbacks. Positions change as others come and go or as the institution changes or as the community changes. Sometimes waiting corrects problems.

But if you have made a serious mistake, then make a change. Even with the most careful effort, you will know less about a new position when you commit to it than you will know after a year in the position. If it becomes necessary, make the change.

In making these decisions, please be good to yourself and to those close to you.

The Role of Clinician

The second role to discuss is that of a clinician. New patients may test you. They want you to have superior knowledge and superior judgment. They want you to listen, show respect, and have empathy, but they also want you to have the professional knowledge that makes it worth consulting you. They want you to have judgment that they can trust. Others can listen, show respect, and have empathy. You are paid for your knowledge and your judgment. Earn your pay.

Listen to your patients with respect, but if you think they are making a wrong health decision, you can say, "That is not what I would recommend."

Explain your thinking. When your patients find that you have thought ethically and humanely about them, they may change their minds. Many of mine did.

In his book, *The Soul of Care,* Arthur Kleinman describes what he learned caring for his wife in her last years. He had not realized the burdens placed on family members or the importance of family members in caring for the sick, the elderly, and the dying. Part of being a good doctor is humility. As doctors, we are a small part of caring for the sick. We are a critical part but still a small part of a great effort.

I once consulted regarding a patient in a nursing home. This patient had a large bedsore across her buttocks extending down into the sacrum. She was in her 50s and had something happen that made her very sick. Her problem might have been an initial infection complicated by Guillain-Barre syndrome, but I never saw the documentation of her diagnosis.

At the low point of her disease, she did not turn herself, nor did any caregiver turn her often enough, so that she developed this terrible bed sore. She had been in a major urban teaching hospital. Because she appeared terminal and unable to tolerate the surgery that would close the ulceration, they sent her to her small hometown to die. In the nursing home, the nurses' aides fed her, cleaned her, and turned her. She healed with no more than this basic good health care. The last time that I saw her she had become strong enough to tolerate a surgical procedure, but she no longer needed it. The bed sore had healed so that it was now covered by scarred skin. The small-town nurses' aides had achieved what the major urban teaching hospital consultants had not.

I congratulated the aides in the nursing home. They deserved every bit of enthusiasm I could muster. We doctors can be quick to criticize and slow to show gratitude. Respect and empathy apply to coworkers as well as to patients. That is basic humanity.

Think about how you will keep up as medicine advances. Learning how to learn is important. In my field of orthopaedics, when major changes in surgery developed, not only did I need to learn new skills, but the team, consisting of the operating room personnel, the nurses, and the physical therapists, had to learn new skills as well. Don't forget your team as things change. Major changes are opportunities for mistakes, so be extra vigilant.

The Role of Teacher

A third role is that of teacher. In addition to Dr. Mankin of the Massachusetts General Hospital, whom I mentioned earlier, another of my favorite professors was Dr. John Hall of Boston Children's Hospital. One of his sayings was, "Good judgment comes from experience. Experience comes from bad judgment."

Dr. Hall gave us residents experience while protecting the patients from bad judgment. He was an exceptional teacher.

The best teacher finds out how far a student has advanced in their learning and then helps them take the next step. Different students have different learning styles—some learn by study at home, some need to watch in a clinical setting, and some learn only by doing. Adapt your teaching to your student's learning style. In a lecture, some students learn from the principles, some from the guidelines, and some from the stories you tell. Consider catering to more than one style.

Avoid shaming a student in public. Criticisms are best done in private, and even then, if you can, sandwich one criticism between two compliments. Praise is a great motivator. Criticism may motivate, but it is more likely to discourage. Criticism carries so much emotional weight that it takes two compliments to begin to balance one criticism.

At their best, teaching hospitals benefit from having students. The presence of students means that fewer diagnoses are missed, more complications are recognized early, attending doctors learn earlier if they have begun to fall behind developments in their field, and the volume of patients supports attending doctors with highly specialized knowledge. When teaching hospitals are at their worst, patients suffer, costs increase, and those with little experience struggle to teach those with less experience. Be careful. As a clinical teacher, you have responsibilities to patients and students. Your responsibility to patients now is to protect them from students' bad judgment. Your responsibility to students is to prepare them for caring for their patients in the future.

Very occasionally, you may have a worrisome student. They are not learning, or their ethics are questionable, or they have significant psychiatric problems. Both humanistic virtue and ethical responsibility to future patients require that you do something. Share your concerns with the student's advisor or others among your colleagues. If others agree, this may be someone who should not graduate from your program. Your program will be judged by those who do graduate. Future generations will depend on your stamps of approval. Be responsible and act when it is the right thing to do.

The Role of Administrator

A fourth role is that of administrator or leader. Effective administrator-leaders will state clear and simple goals and then give those under them the freedom to accomplish the goals. Adhere to the goals yourself—you will be watched. Monitor each employee's performance. Employees want to know that what they do is important enough for you to pay attention. They also perform better if they know that you will notice.

Consider meeting once a year, one-on-one, with key personnel. In these meetings, seek information as well as give it. Those whom you lead may know before you do what they need to do a better job for your unit or when a problem is developing. Some corporations include what are called "skip-level interviews." A manager meets annually not only with those at the level that reports directly to the manager, but also skips a level to interview a few of those at lower levels. In my field of orthopaedics, the physical therapists knew who the questionable surgeons were even when the department chief did not. Had the chief done skip-level interviews with a few physical therapists each year, he would have known.

Write annual reports, even if no one else requests them and they go into a folder that no one but you sees. Review the good and the not so good of the past year. Consider plans and concerns for the next year. Recording this thinking once a year means that you have done it once a year.

If you need to criticize or discipline someone, do it in private, perhaps with a third person as a witness. Start by seeking more information about the issue. You may have misinterpreted the situation. If you haven't, explain your views. If possible, sandwich your critical comment between two complimentary comments, as you would with a student. Explain what you expect and how you will follow up. Do not expect an apology or resolution at this meeting. You are not looking for an apology and you won't yet have the resolution. You are looking for a change. You will know later that the meeting was successful if you see improvement.

Pay attention to morale. Meet regularly with your staff. Seek their thoughts before making any significant changes. One able leader told me that he discussed decisions democratically and then made decisions autocratically. Have your staff meet for social activities, such as a December party or a summer outing. Give bonuses when appropriate and if the organization allows it.

Do what you can to retain staff—recruiting replacements takes time, and the new person will be inefficient for months after they start. A little effort at retention replaces a great deal of effort at recruitment and retraining.

I believe that the best leaders are humane. I believe that the best leaders are responsible, respectful, and empathetic.

The Role of Researcher

A fifth role is that of the researcher. My primary interest has always been in clinical medicine, so I will tell you about one of the two 2023 Nobel Prize in Medicine winners, Katalin Kariko. She was born in Hungary in 1955 and trained in biology there, progressing to a Ph.D. She worked in a laboratory in Hungary, but that laboratory lost its funding. In 1985, she came to this country with her husband and daughter. After a tumultuous four years working in three other places, she found a position at the University of Pennsylvania.

Part of the tumult was the negative attitude of her first boss. She worked on messenger RNA and how it could be used pharmacologically. A paper describing her key discoveries was rejected by *Nature* and by *Science*. At the time, established researchers believed that messenger RNA research would not be productive. Kariko was unable to get grants. She was rejected for tenure at the University of Pennsylvania. Industry showed more interest, and when the COVID epidemic occurred, Moderna and Pfizer used her work and that of her research colleague, Drew Weissman, to produce vaccines. That led to their Nobel Prizes.

Research is a tough way to make a living. Researchers live from grant to grant. To an outsider like me, success appears to come from learning the right techniques, studying the right problems, the intensity of a researcher's interest, and obtaining results at the right time to have them applied.

One of the new techniques of this time is CRISPR to modify nucleic acids. Those who learn this new technique are finding many ways to apply it. Older technologies have already been used often enough so that mastering them offers fewer new opportunities. The latest technologies tend to be the most productive.

Studying the right problem at the right time helps. Dr. Kariko was ahead of her time so she could not get tenure, but she had selected a problem that could be solved, and she was right that the solution would prove useful. For those ahead of their time, it helps to be only a little ahead.

The intensity of interest helps. Dr. Kariko, it is reported, read widely and thought deeply about her work. Winston Churchill once said, "Success is the ability to go from one failure to another with no loss of enthusiasm." Dr. Kariko persisted in the face of repeated set-backs.

Researchers have not always been ethical in their treatment of animals and have not always respected the autonomy of human subjects. Relationships between researchers have not always been humane and ethical. We hear of men who took the credit for discoveries made by women. Should you choose a research career, do not forget ethics and humanity.

Research can be exceptionally rewarding. I cannot imagine what Kariko and Weissman felt after their work limited the suffering from the COVID epidemic. One of my mentors described clinical medicine as retail, helping people one by one. Research is helping wholesale, delivering help to all of society.

· · · · ·

Which should you choose—clinical work, teaching, administration, or research? As with the choice of specialty, consider what you value, what you can do well, and what you enjoy. Then make a choice and concentrate, for it is only with concentration in a single area that you will do your best work.

But then, life can take unexpected turns, and when it does, you may need to change roles. Consider not focusing too narrowly during training. For each of us, there are many paths to satisfaction. If you find that one path is blocked, look for another that you can follow. If you need to change, don't obsess by looking back over what might have been. Think about any lessons you can learn and then turn your attention and your energy to moving forward along a new path. Those before you have found satisfaction in all the roles we have considered—clinician, teacher, leader, and researcher. Don't despair. If, like Dr. Kariko, events force you to change positions, change.

The Chinese have a saying: "Sometimes when you lose, you win." Dr. Kariko lost several times. She always found a new path until one led to a Nobel Prize. You don't have to win that big, but you can find satisfaction along many paths.

Chapter Twelve

Concluding Thoughts

As I wrote this book, I thought of the story of the blind men learning about an elephant by touch. The one who felt the trunk thought the elephant was like a snake, the one who felt a leg thought the elephant was like a tree, the one who felt the flank thought that the elephant was like a wall, and the one who felt the tail thought the elephant was like a brush.

As I began, I thought the elephant that I was palpating was a humanistic or ethical elephant. I may have found only parts of the beast. At times, I may have wandered to another elephant so that the atheistic humanistic elephant was a different elephant from the theistic humanistic elephant. Then I wandered off to palpate a beast that was not an elephant at all, but something involving matters of money, cultures or careers.

In short, this book may contain too little or too much. It does contain too little, for there is more for you to learn about every subject in it. It does contain too much, for it wandered beyond my main topics. What is just right is providing you with an introduction to ethics, humanism and other important matters at the beginning of your medical career. You will learn more about each of these matters with time and experience. May you enjoy, as my classmates and I have enjoyed, what we believe to be the best career in the world: being a medical doctor.

Notes About the Bibliography

A recent president of Harvard resigned in part because she had been careless in citing sources. That gave me pause, for I was well into the preparation of this book when she resigned. I had been relaxed, perhaps too relaxed, thinking of this book as avuncular advice rather than original scholarly work. By the standards that had been applied to the Harvard president, I have been careless.

Perhaps I can be excused for not recording my oldest sources. This book reflects a lifetime of experiences, during which I have misplaced or discarded my college ethics text and forgotten the author's name. Likewise for my college economics text, except that I remember the last name of the author, which was Samuelson. His first name was Paul, which I had forgotten but it was easy to look up. Almost 20 years after finishing college I read a book with the concept of you, me, and us and promptly discarded it, thinking that I would never need to look at it again.

Less excusable was my neglect to record the dates and titles of the Wikipedia searches last year when I looked for the oaths in chapter six and for the details of almost every biographical sketch in the book. When I did go back to Wikipedia in a search for the reference I had seen to the editor of Aristotle's *Ethics*, I could not find it. The site may already have been altered. By luck, I found the book itself on one of my shelves. I can only hope that the other Wikipedia references that I used have not been deleted.

I have omitted footnote references in the text, thinking that most readers would not use them and would find them a distraction. There will be readers who will want to check my sources or read further on a topic. Hopefully they will find their ways easily enough from the text through the bibliography to the important sources.

Please assume that any important concept or philosophy in this book is something that I learned from someone else, whether I remember who that someone else was or not. The personal stories in the book are original, of course. They would not belong in a more scholarly book. They are more appropriate in a relaxed book like this one.

Bibliography

Aristotle, translated by David Ross, with an introduction and notes by Lesley Brown, *The Nichomachean Ethics,* Oxford University Press, Oxford, England, 1980.

Aristotle, translated with an introduction and notes by H. C. Lawson-Tancred, *The Art of Rhetoric,* Penguin Books, London, England, 1991.

Bakewell, Sarah, *Humanly Possible,* Penguin Press, New York, N. Y., 2023.

Beauchamp, Tom L., and James F. Childress, *Principles of Biomedical Ethics,* 8th ed., Oxford University Press, Oxford, England, 2019.

Berne, Eric, *Games People Play,* Ballentine Publishing Group, New York, N. Y. 1964.

Carter, Zachary D., *The Price of Peace: Money, Democracy, and the Life of John Maynard Keynes,* Random House, New York, 2020.

Copson, Andrew, and Roberts, Alice, *The Little Book of Humanism,* Piatkus (of Little Brown Book Group), London, England, 2020.

Epictetus, *The Encheiridion,* in *Epictetus: The Discourses as Reported by Arrian, The Manual, and Fragments,* vol. 2, Harvard University Press, Cambridge, MA, 1928, reprinted by Franklin Classics Trade Press, 2022.

Erikson, Erik, *Childhood and Society,* W. H. Norton and Co., New York, N. Y., 1950, 1993.

Fadiman, Anne, *The Spirit Catches You and You Fall Down,* Farrar, Straus, and Giroux, New York, N. Y., 1997.

Kidder, Tracy, *Mountains Beyond Mountains,* Random House, 2009.

Kidder, Tracy, *Rough Sleepers,* Random House, 2024.

Kristeller, Paul Oskar, *Humanism,* Minerva 16(4):586-595, Winter, 1978.

Lamont, Corliss, *The Philosophy of Humanism,* 8th ed., Humanist Press, Washington, D. C., 2001.

Mill, John Stuart, edited by Mark Philp and Frederick Rosen, *On Liberty, Utilitarianism, and Other Essays,* Oxford University Press, Oxford, England, 2015.

Newby, Eric, *A Short Walk in the Hindu Kush,* Harper Press, 1956.

Robinson, George, *Essential Judaism,* Atria Paperback (Simon and Schuster), New York, NY, 2000 and 2016.

Rosenbaum, Lisa, *On Calling—From Privileged Professionals to Cogs of Capitalism?* New England Journal of Medicine 390(5):471-475, Feb. 1, 2024.

Szasz, T. S., and Hollender, Marc H., *A Contribution to the Philosophy of Medicine; the Basic Models of the Doctor-Patient Relationship,* AMA Arch Intern Med, May 1956, 95 (5):585-592.

Theroux, Paul, *On the Plain of Snakes,* Mariner Books, 2020.

Thubron, Colin, *The Amur River: Between Russia and China,* Harper, 2021.

Biographical Note

I grew up in the small town of Merrill, Wisconsin, where my father was a family physician. I went to Carleton College and Harvard Medical School, followed by two years of general surgery training at Stanford University and three and a half years in the orthopaedic residency at Harvard. Because of the Vietnam war, all of us from my medical school class of 1967 spent time either in the military or in alternative federal service. I interrupted residency training to spend two years in the United States Air Force, stationed in western South Dakota. Our base hospital served both a military population and the indigenous Americans on the nearby Pine Ridge Reservation. Later, during my residency, I spent a three-month elective with Project Hope at the University of the West Indies Hospital in Kingston, Jamaica.

After completing my orthopaedic residency, I worked at Northwestern University Medical School, at the Beth Israel Hospital in Boston, in a private practice in central Massachusetts (Central Orthopaedics), and, for the last eight years of my career, at the UMass Chan Medical School. While at Northwestern, I was first author of a paper describing a safe zone to guide insertion of the cup or socket side of a total hip replacement. That paper has had over 2,000 citations. I understand that the safe zone is used now by robots as they are introduced into total hip replacement surgery.

Including summers as a student in laboratories, I have had experiences as a student, as a clinician in several settings (teaching hospital, private hospital, military hospital, Veteran's Administration hospital, and third-world hospital), as a teacher, as a researcher, and as an administrator running a small private practice.

Opinions and Acknowledgments

The opinions expressed in this book are my own and have not been approved by Harvard, the Humanism in Medicine Initiative, or by anyone else.

There have been many influences on my thinking. They began in my childhood, with my mother, Beryl Nelson Lewinnek, R.N., who first told me a concept of a good doctor, and my father, Walter Lewinnek, M.D., a family doctor who was a role model of responsibility, respect, and empathy. During summers in college, I worked in a laboratory at the University of Minnesota under James Pierce, M.D. He made the comment about research being a way to help people wholesale. I remain awed by his scholarship, productivity, and humanity.

Three physician authors who are not listed in the bibliography deserve mention. They are Jerome Groopman, Oliver Sachs and Atul Gawande. I have not listed their works in the bibliography since, in the text, I referred to none of them. Should you choose to do so, you may find as much pleasure in reading them as I did.

Beyond these, I am in debt to all who have trained me, to colleagues and friends who have enriched my life, and especially to my significant other, Susan Tarrant. Susan made great contributions to the writing of this book with her editing skills, her knowledge of medical ethics, and her encouraging words. My son, David Lewinnek, and my daughter, Karen Lewinnek Teelin, M.D., made important suggestions. I have been helped by Winslow Green, M.D.; Thomas Gutheil, M.D.; Larry Kadish, M.D.; Gordon Weir, M.D.; Young Kim, M.D.; Micayla Flores, medical student; and Tom Hunt, retired minister. These individuals reviewed drafts, offered suggestions, provided encouragement, and corrected as many errors as possible. Any errors that remain are my own responsibility.

www.ingramcontent.com/pod-product-compliance
Lightning Source LLC
Chambersburg PA
CBHW020437220526
45464CB00002B/741